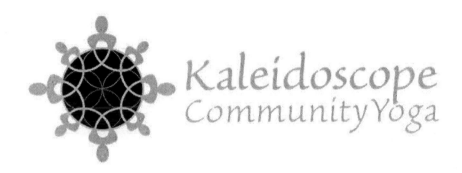

Book 1: the first 108 poses

(art of connecting series)

Kaleidoscope Community Yoga: Book 1: The first 108 poses
(The art of connecting series)

© 2012 Lo Nathamundi.
Infinite Designs Publishing.
Printed in the United States of America.

FIRST EDITION
FOURTH PRINTING

Printed on the Espresso Book Machine at Powell's Books in Portland, Oregon.

Book cover design by Desirae Hill
Author photo on back cover by Zeck Koa

ISBN: 978-0-692-01841-5
Library of Congress number 2012944622

Body text font: Calibri

info@kldyoga.org
loswirlingwaters@gmail.com

Namaste.

GRATITUDE.

It all starts with gratitude.

Heart-felt thank you's to my mother, my father, my brother, and all of my teachers, mentors, friends, and relations. My ancestors, spirit guides, and the divine inner wisdom within all of us.

Thank you.

James Bauckman for video, Desirae Hill for graphic, web, and logo design. Jenny Macke and Presence Studio, Justin Bilancieri and Café Bloom, Alborz Monjazeb and the Majestic, for providing studio space.

Thank you.

Teddy Anderson, Andy Bronson, Stephen Bruno, Jaime Hernandez, John Hogl, Jorge Lausell, Alex Peregrina, and all the photographers, amateur and professional, who have taken photographs of the yoga project.

Thank you.

Becca Barbanell ("Dreamyball Dang"), Sam Bliss, Misty Flowers, Jordan Goldberg, Mehdi Makraz, Burke Mulvany, and anyone else who has ever played music for the project.

Thank you.

Everyone who served on the Kaleidoscope Crew during the first two years: Danielle AhMaiua, Brian Anderson, Jill Beringer, Sarah Bolivar, Erica ("Lilly") May Cary, Heather Comforto, Bryan Givens, Carolyn Hallett, Desirae Hill, Larry Hurvitz, Nolan Hoppe-Leonard, Mehdi Makraz, Alborz Monjazeb, Lo Nathamundi, Carol Ouellette, Alex Peregrina, Caitlin Quigley, Danny Ray, Dannie Soloff, Jill Sturdevant, Molly Van Hart, Aaron Webb, Noah Young.

Thank you.

And especially...
Jill Noelani Sturdevant, muse, companion, lover, partner, magic fern, and constant source of support to both me and the yoga project since its birth.
Co-author and co-inspiration of many of the poses in a way that is way beyond what words could ever describe.

Thank you.

Teachers, mentors, friends, colleagues, students, helpers, and inspirations who deserve special mention: Ingela Abbot, Adam Ross Alkire, Chipp Allard, David Anders ("Majnun"), Brian Anderson, Jane Armstrong, Sus Arnhart, Suki Aufhauser, Max Barahona, Liz Bart, Bruce Bartlett, Robert Bates, Cody Beebe, Tammy Bennett, Devin Beu, Ken Bothman, Kelsey Bowen, Danny Bronny, Matthew Brouwer, Eric Brown, Tshombe Brown, Bob Cantley, Jesse Charette, Sara Charette, Alona Christman, Matt Christman, Brendan Clark, Andrew Connor, Casey Connor, Leslie Conton, Cate Cook, Julia Crouch, Judith Culver, Christian Czingula, Tana Dasilva, Antonio Diaz, Clara Dominguez, Susan D'onofrio, Stephanie Dougherty, Deborah Dove, Jordan Edwards, Richard Lotni Elm-Hill, Link ("Littlepaw") Falsetto, Jeri Ferguson, CC Fish, Matt Fogarty, Aimee Trebon Frazier, Paige Fredlund, Karl Freske, Stan Freske, Nancy Garing, Sylvie Gendron, Alexander Georgeakopoulos, Joel Gillman, Bryan Givens, Sheila Goldsmith, Susan Grace, Joules Graves, Ashaman Gray, Lisa Greenacre, Laura Greenwood, Meena Harlow, Heather Haugland, John Hawkins, Chad Helder, Olivier Hetzel, Joel Hirsch, Harrison Holtzman-Knott, Leif Honstad, Spruce Horowitz, Jill Hummelstein, Summer Huntington, Laura Husbeck, Lisa Iversen, Michael Jaross, Keith Johnson, Aard Jordan, Mialee Jose, Chikeola Karimou, Renee Kennedy, Michael Knudsen, Ruby Koa, Susan Kocen, Georgia Komons, Dave Koshinz, Alyssa Krist, Pam Kuntz, Steven Lacroix, Mark Lakeman, Kate LaSpina, Laura Lavigne, Daniel Lebedies, Namgyl Lhamo, Paul Li, Michael Light, Gayle Livingston, Thomas Lucklum, Melanie Lum, Jenny Macke, Rachael Maddalena, Augustine Magdalene, Carla Mangione, Auguste Manne, Andrew Marks, Emily Marston, Charles Mattoon, Mateo Mblem, Lindsey McGuirk, Austin McHugh, Don Meneely, Rick Merrill, Nancy Metcalf, Jane Midget, Paul Millage, Arny Mindell, Stephanie Mohler, Alborz Monjazeb, Jane Gray Morris, Della Moustachella, Burke Mulvany, Hernan Neira, Frank Nelson, Scot Nichols, Paul Norlen, Chris O'Dell, Dan O'Donnell, Cheryl Ogden, James Rian O'Keefe, Heidi Ormbrek, Guy Ortiz, Bill Ottercrans, Densley Palmer, Brian Patterson, Kraig ("Bopi") Patterson, Aleksandr Peikrshvilli, Alex Peregrina, Jan Peters, Greg Peterson, Karen Piccone, Skeeter Pilarski, Bill Pinar, Alden Ramel, Alex Ramel, Violeta Ramsay, Dan Ratayczak, Lauron Ray, Alicia Recart, Mario Recart, Puanani Reid, Tim Reid, Michal Retter, Enrique Perojo Revilla, RJ Rex, Christina Reyes, Shola Angela Ricco, Peter Richardson, Edgar de Los Rios, Amy Robinson, Matt Robinson, Elizabeth Ruff, Richard Sands, Marjorie Scarlett, James Weston Schaberg, Marlene Schenter, Aldo Schipper, August Scialfa, John Seaman, Lee Seaman, Alan Seid, Wailana Simcock, Lillian Soderman, Dannie Soloff, Daniel Solomons, Chris Spilker, Gabe Springsnow, Aron Stanley, Abby Staten, Rob Staveland, Chris Strelau, Meg Sutton, Barb Swanson-Fisher, Brigitte Sztab, Bryan Thomas, Seth Tichenor,

Jessica Tokarchuk, Arisana Tolomei, Suzanne Tom, Stephen Trinkaus, James Ray Turner, Sara Vandepas, Will Van Inwagen, Mitch Vega, Rose Vogel, Katie Wall, Adam Ward, Andy Wargo, Dylan Warnberg, Corey Warren, Lise Waugh, Denise Webber, Nancy Welch, Christina Wienhold, Stacey Williams, Lee Willis, Drew Winsor, Robert Woodford, Maya Wright, Leilani Zimmerman, and many more, and more to come.

Thank you.

One love. Infinite designs.

A few words about the photos in this manual:

Thank you to everyone who has participated in the poses over the years and shared themselves with others through photos.

While every reasonable effort was made to choose photos demonstrating proper alignment, please know that we make no claims as to the perfection of alignment of every person in every photo. Many of the photos shown are candid shots of people with varying levels of yoga experience sharing yoga together in the park. As such, the alignment is not always "perfect." These are extraordinary "ordinary" people on an extraordinary path of growth. They are snapshots of living, growing human beings. Their growth is a process. Which is its own perfect "imperfection."

Every reasonable effort was made to catalog everyone who showed up in the photos and everyone who helped take the photos. For those who only came once, or are blurry, or are in the background, or somehow didn't get listed in the pose credits or photo credits section at the back of the book, all apologies. Sincere apologies to anyone whose name we missed.

Thank you.

TABLE OF CONTENTS

DEDICATION

This book is dedicated to all students of collective yoga, and to the growth of shared yoga practice as a common human activity. To anyone who has ever joined us for a pose, especially the ones who were nervous or afraid to. To a vision of all of humanity, peacefully, harmoniously sharing touch and contact and connection.

May this book be a gift towards that purpose.

So far as I know, it is the first and only book of its kind. It is the first and only book devoted solely to mapping, discussing, and presenting a comprehensive system of intertwined, interconnected yoga poses for groups, made available to the general public.

And now you are a part of it.

With much love,

Logermund Nathamundi

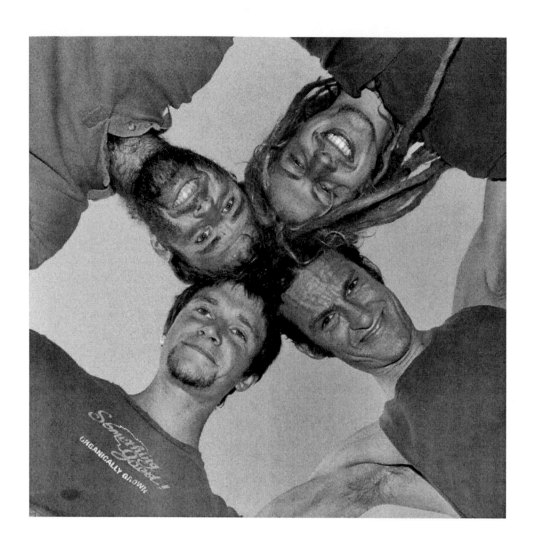

Hello, and welcome to community yoga.

Kaleidoscope /kəˈlaɪdəˌskoʊp/

[Gk. *kalos*, beautiful + *eidos*, shape, form + *skopein*, to see]

1. A toy, consisting of a tube with mirrors, and small pieces of colored glass or other material, whose reflections produce an endless variety of moving patterns and geometric shapes.
2. A style of community yoga, similar to the toy, where participants share their energy, and make an endless variety of geometrical shapes and patterns together, serving as mirrors for one another's alignment.
3. A social or spiritual practice of the same.

As in **kaleidoscope yoga**, or **kaleidoscope community yoga**.

"Wow, what an amazingly fun **Kaleidoscope Community Yoga** jam!" – typical Kaleidoscope Community Yoga participant

Entry taken from p. 108 of the LOED (Lo's English Dictionary)

Community /kəˈmyunɪti/

[Old Fr. *communité*, Latin *communitas, cum*, with, together + *munus*, gift]

1. A tribe, group, collective.
2. Sharing, union, synergy.
3. A feeling of well-being that comes from sharing.

As in **community-style**, **feeling of community**, or **community living**.

"Wow, it feels so good to be a part of this **community**!" – typical community member

Entry taken from p. 24 of the LOED (Lo's English Dictionary)

Yoga /ˈyoʊɡə/

[Skt. *yeug*, yoke, union, joining]

1. A series of physical exercises designed to bring health to the body, peace to the mind, and enlightenment to the soul.
2. A practice of meditation.
3. A path of spiritual growth.
4. A path of social or spiritual service.

As in **bhakti yoga**, or **hatha yoga**.

"Wow, **yoga** has made such a difference in my life!" – typical yoga student

Entry taken from p. 777 of the LOED (Lo's English Dictionary)

INTRODUCTION

What is Kaleidoscope Community Yoga?

Kaleidoscope Community Yoga is a new type of social activity, and a new way to practice yoga. A new way to relate to one another. A new form of group process.

Kaleidoscope Community Yoga is a specific style or system of practicing yoga as a group. During a typical class or session, often called a 'jam,' there is a teacher, sometimes called the 'facilitator,' or 'guide,' or 'caller,' and the group, or students, or community. The teacher begins the session, shares a warm-up, and then leads the group through a series of group yoga poses and sequences. The facilitator may also call for requests or open the process up to the creativity of the group. At the end of the session, the facilitator conducts a closing of some kind.

Think of it as square dancing meets yoga, or having fun while mapping the collective human yoga genome.

PREFACE

Kaleidoscope Yoga: The universal heart and the individual self.

We, as humanity, make up together a mosaic of beautiful colors and shapes that can harmoniously play together in endless combinations. We are an ever-changing play of shape and form. A kaleidoscope consists of a tube (or container), mirrors, pieces of glass (or beads or precious stones), sunlight, and someone to turn it and observe and enjoy the forms. Metaphorically, perhaps the sun represents the divine light, or spark of life, within all of us. The mirrors represent our ability to serve as mirrors for one another and each other's alignment, reflecting sides of ourselves that we may not have been aware of. The tube (or container) is the practice of community yoga. We, as human beings, are the glass, the beads, the precious stones. The facilitator is the person turning the Kaleidoscope, initiating the changing patterns. And the resulting beauty of the shapes? Well, that's for everyone to enjoy...

Coming into a practice and an energy field of community yoga over and over, is a practice of returning, again and again, to the present moment, to the person in front of you, to the people around you, to your body, to others' bodies, to your energy, to others' energy, to your breath, to others' breath.

Like the ancient Hindu dictum "I am that" (tat twam asi), community yoga practice can help us, in a very real, practical, grounded, felt, somatic way, to identify and be in harmony with all that is around us, which includes all of our fellow human beings. We are all multiple selves. We are all infinite. We are all universal selves. We are all unique expressions of the universal heart and universal energy. We are all the universal self. We are all one another. And we are all also unique specific individuals. And to the extent that we practice this, somatically, we become more and more comfortable and fluid with this larger, more cosmic, more inter-related reality. We see and feel and breathe ourselves, more and more, as the open movement of energy, as open somatic possibility. As energy and breath. This is one of the many benefits of a community yoga practice. Kaleidoscope shows us, in a very practical way, how to allow universal patterns of wisdom and interconnectedness to filter through us. Eventually, the bones become mere anchors, reference points for the structures of open movement...

One of the most interesting paradoxes I have encountered during my involvement with the community yoga project (and it is one that I have felt again and again, too many times to count) is the paradox that many of the most infinite, universal forms have come to me in a place of absolute solitude, silence, deep aloneness or meditation. And, similarly, conversely and complimentarily, (best not to get stuck on the words) I have often found myself in the midst of a huge crowd or group of people of seamlessly flowing forms, and felt simultaneously, in addition to the group energy, the group shape, and the group awareness, myself as a very cleanly and clearly defined, very particular, individual self. These moments and discoveries and journeys of group awareness, in addition to the sense of cosmic expansion, have also clarified more strongly my sense of a very specific, rooted, personal self.

The more deeply I dive into the universal heart, the more clearly I see my own place in it. And the more deeply I tune in and connect with my own true personal self, the more open and available I am to a larger, more universal self.

We are both, universal heart and universal self. Individual heart and individual self. We are, or have the capacity for, or however you choose to put it, simultaneous layers of awareness. Learning to feel and navigate and mediate between these different kinds and layers of awareness is one of the great joys of Kaleidoscope Community Yoga, and of life in general.

Come join us, and see what that feels like, in your body, again and again.

THE POSES

Beginning (Levels 1-3)
1 sequence, 18 poses (#'s 1-18)

1. silence (1)
2. standing prayer (1)
3. om circle (1)
4. name circle (1)

5-9. CLASSIC SEQUENCE #1: opening warrior circle (3)
5. warrior I circle (3)
6. warrior II circle (3)
7. reverse warrior circle (3)
8. triangle pose circle (3)
9. infallible warrior dominoes (3)

10. earth, heart, sky (2)
11. partner handshakes (1)
12. partner bow (1)
13. partner hip sink (3)
14. group child's pose (3)
15. group ear massage (2)
16. standing prayer hands heart circle (1)
17. group spiral shavasana circle (3)
18. seated prayer hands heart circle (1)

Intermediate (Levels 4-6)
2 sequences, 36 poses (#'s 19-54)

19. hamstring square (4)
20. trivial pursuit pie carousel spin (4)
21. trivial pursuit pie straddle forward fold (5)
22. paper doll parade (5)
23. group tree pose (5)
24. group spinal twist (5)
25. dancer bigtop (5)
26. dancer directional circle (6)
27. shared 3rd eye bow (5)
28. prayer hand flower (5)
29. sunflower backbend (6)
30. ski-jumper (6)
31. partner boat splits (6)
32. 3-8 person boat (6)
33. sidestretch paper foldouts (6)
34. pinwheel (5)
35. ship at sea (5)
36. caterpillar east and west (6)

37-41. CLASSIC SEQUENCE #2: butterflies (6)
37. butterfly twist line (6)
38. butterfly neck rest (6)
39. butterfly breathing (5)
40. butterfly side-stretches (6)
41. butterfly tabletop press (6)

42. partner straddle see-saw line (6)
43. grass-in-the-wind (6)

44-48. CLASSIC SEQUENCE #3: baddha konasana clover (6)
44. baddha konasana clover forward fold (6)
45. baddha konasana clover hands to knees (5)
46. baddha konasana clover huddle (6)

47. baddha konasana clover stir the pot (5)
48. baddha konasana clover eggbeaters (5)

49. ballet leg lifts (6)
50. eagle arms line (6)
51. eagle arms cosmic spiral squawk walk in a circle (6)
52. elephant trunks, elephant ankles (6)
53. pigeon circle (6)
54. pigeon huddle (6)

Advanced (Levels 7-9)
3 sequences, 54 Poses (#'s 55-108)

55. skydive circle (7)
56. diamond dogs (7)
57. side dogs (7)
58. dandelion (7)
59. spider (7)
60. short grass, tall grass (7)

61-67. CLASSIC SEQUENCE #4: partner warrior fractal (7)
61. partner warrior I (7)
62. partner warrior II (7)
63. partner reverse warrior (7)
64. partner straddle hang (7)
65. partner ankle grab (7)
65. partner same side twist (8)
66. partner opposite side twist (8)
67. partner triangle pose (7)

68. side-reclining buddha wheel (7)
69. baddha konasana clover thai massage twist assist (7)
70. baddha konasana clover thai massage backwalk (7)
71. dog-back (7)
72. 4-hand massage for child's pose (7)
73. dog-back skydive (7)
74. crab cross lift (7)
75. crab cross tetrahedron lift (8)
76. acro-on-the boat deck (7)
77. shaolin horse hamstrings (7)
78. zipper legs arm-wrestler leanaway (7)
79. zipper legs crab-lift (8)
80. pigeon pairs (7)
81. air traffic control (7)
82. jellyfish hip and sacrum massage collective (7)
83. lunge circle (7)

84. pyramid circle (8)
85. reclining hero family takes the train (7)
86. grass-in-the-wind hexagon (8)
87. trillium reclining heroes and heroines (8)
88. yin/ yang straddle plow, seated straddle (8)
89. grounded swaying palms (8)
90. standing back-to-back lift (8)

91-97. CLASSIC SEQUENCE #5: legagon (7)
91. legagon (7)
92. legagon huddle (7)
93. legagon leanback (8)
94. legagon cosmic spiral leanaway (7)
95. legagon hand-to-foot twist (7)
96. legagon hand-to-hand twist (8)
97. supported legagon (7)

98-101. CLASSIC SEQUENCE #6: sloth family portrait (8)
98. sloth family portrait (8)
99. loving sloth family portrait (8)
100. ambitious sloth family portrait (8)
101. sloths play peek-a-boo (9)

102. handstand pillars (8)
103. lumberjack free-hang (9)
104. lumberjack chiropractor (9)
105. lumberjack ankle grab (9)
106. humaneering (partner climb-around) (9)
107. diamond dogs with partial (1-person) levitation (9)
108. davinci's counterbalance (9)

<u>Beginning (Levels 1-3)</u>

Introductory poses are a fun and easy way for anyone to get involved. They are good for warming up, closing, and large, inexperienced, or unfamiliar groups. There is no or very little weight-sharing between participants. Many of the poses in this group are simple standing or seated positions.

1. silence (1)

DESCR: Participants stand in a circle, facing the center. Feet together, hands to heart center. Eyes closed.
CAUTIONS:
CALLING: "You can come into a circle, with your feet together, and hands together at heart center. You can close your eyes if you like. Just noticing your breath. Maybe feeling some gratitude or setting an intention for your practice."
NOTES:

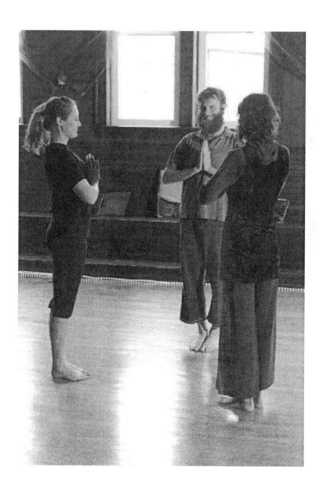

2. standing prayer (1)

DESCR: Participants stand in a circle, facing the center. Feet together, hands to heart center. Eyes closed.
CAUTIONS:
CALLING: "You can come into a circle, with your feet together, and hands together at heart center. You can close your eyes if you like. Noticing your breath. Saying or feeling a prayer or some gratitude."
NOTES:

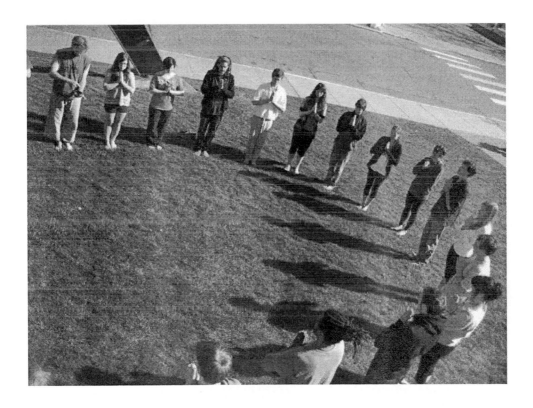

3. om circle (1)

DESCR: Participants stand in a circle, facing the center. Feet together, hands to heart center.
CAUTIONS:
CALLING: "Okay, everyone, we're going to OM together 3 times. Take a nice big inhale. OMMMM. [pause] OMMMM. [pause] OMMMM."
NOTES:
VARIATIONS: Chanting, devotional singing, 'Moo circle.'

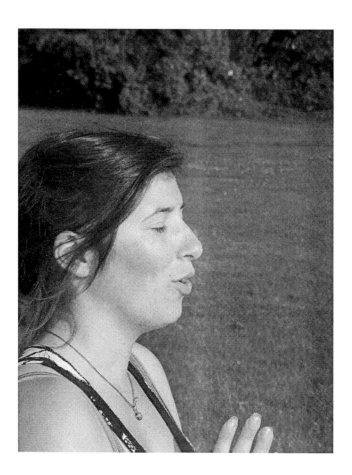

4. name circle (1)

DESCR: Participants stand in a circle, facing the center. Each person shares their name with the group.
CAUTIONS:
CALLING: "So we're just going to do a quick name circle, so we know who we're doing yoga with today. I'll start. My name is..."
NOTES:
VARIATIONS: Just for fun, go back around the circle in the opposite direction, and have people say their names backwards.

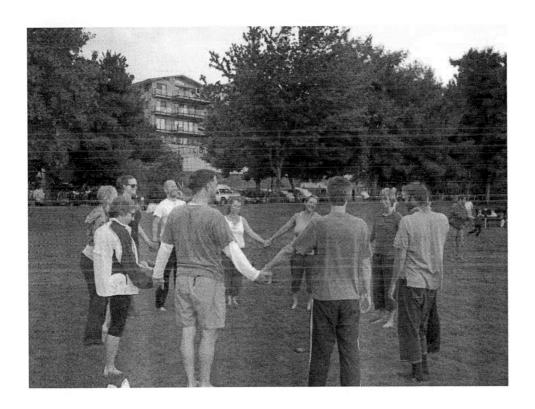

5-9. CLASSIC SEQUENCE #1: opening warrior circle (3)

5. warrior I circle
6. warrior II circle
7. reverse warrior circle
8. triangle pose circle
9. infallible warrior dominoes

DESCR: Participants stand in a circle, shoulder-to-shoulder, facing in toward the center. WI, WII, reverse warrior, WII, triangle pose, hand to neighbor's shoulder, hand to sky, repeat, hand-to-hip, back up to WII, step to middle, repeat on other side.
CAUTIONS:
CALLING: "Starting feet together, hands together. Let's all step our right foot back, coming into Warrior I. Exhale, arms down to Warrior II. Front knee over the ankle. Turn the front hand over so the palm faces the sky. Inhale, back to reverse warrior. Breathing here. Exhale, forward to warrior II. Inhale, lengthen the spine, straighten the front leg, and then exhale, sweeping down into triangle pose, bottom hand on the ankle or shin, top hand to the sky. Breath here. Exhale, top hand gently to neighbor's shoulder in front of you, it makes a circle all the way around, inhale top hand to the sky. Exhale, top hand to neighbor's shoulder. Inhale, top hand to the sky. Exhale, top hand to your own hip. Inhale, lift to warrior II, step your back foot forward and we'll try it again on the other side. Let's all step our left foot back, coming into Warrior I..."
NOTES:

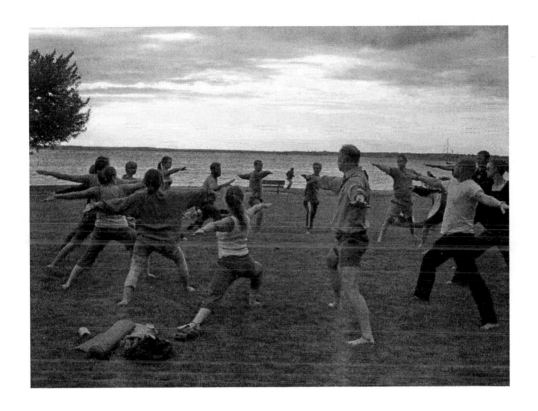

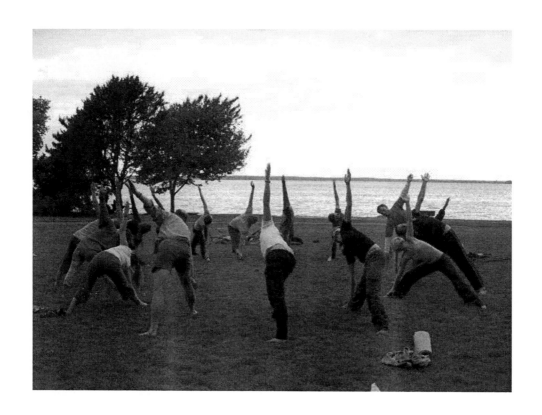

10. earth, heart, sky (2)

DESCR: Participants stand in a circle, facing the center. Feet together, hands to neighbor's shoulders.
CAUTIONS:
CALLING: "Starting with hands to neighbor's shoulders, you can reach around behind a little further to what we call the second neighbors' hands, interlacing your fingers with their fingers. Then, lower this 'rope' of the arms down to heart level. Keeping the hands together, inhale up, hands towards the sky, exhale down, forward fold, hands toward the earth. Inhale up, towards the sky. Exhale, behind."
NOTES:
VARIATIONS: Tussle your neighbor's hair on the way up. When you get to the bottom, gently nuzzle neighbors' foreheads on either side with your shared hands.
SLANG NAMES: "What breathes up, must breathe down."
RELATED POSES: See also, pose #89, grounded swaying palms.

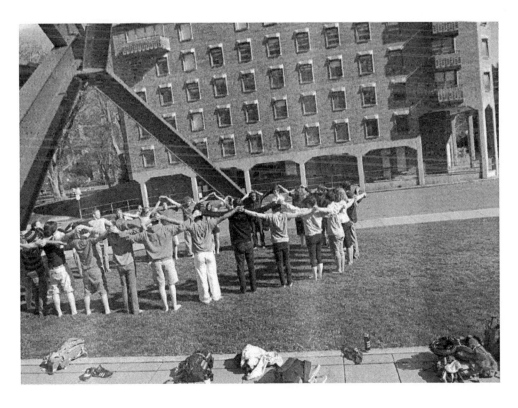

11. partner handshakes (right-right and left-left) (1)

DESCR: Participants stand facing one another, in one or more lines.
CAUTIONS:
CALLING: "Stand facing your partner. Reach out and shake partner's hand. Give them a smile. Introduce yourself if you don't know them, give them a familiar smile if you do. Now switch. Shake the other hand, just to keep it even."
NOTES:
VARIATIONS: Pattycake, jellyfish handshake, secret handshakes, etc.

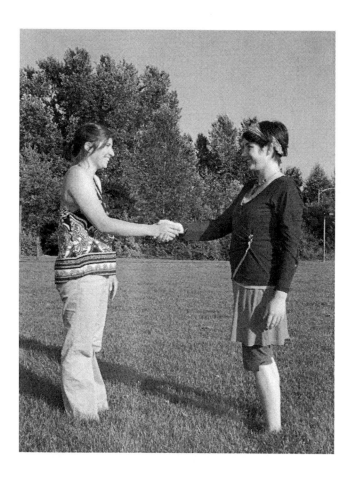

12. partner bow (1)

DESCR: Participants stand facing one another, in one or more lines. Feet together. Bow.
CAUTIONS:
CALLING: "Stand facing your partner. Feet together. Gently bow to your partner, acknowledging them and honoring them and the yoga that you will share together."
NOTES:

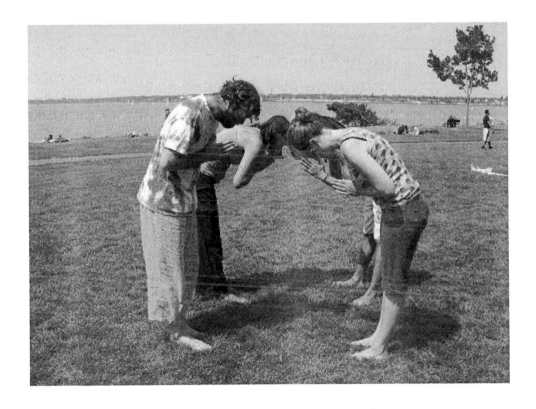

13. partner hip sink (3)

DESCR: Participants stand facing one another, in one or more lines.
CAUTIONS:
CALLING: "Standing, facing your partner. Feet straight under the hips. Find partner's hands or wrists. Fold in half by sinking your weight back at the hips."
NOTES: Once you have a good grip, go ahead and really sink into it. If you're flexible, you may be surprised to see how low and how far back you can go.
VARIATIONS: Hands to neighbor's shoulders.

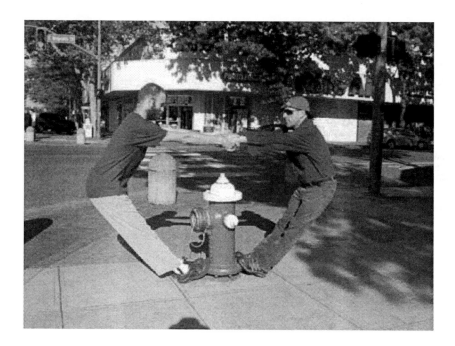

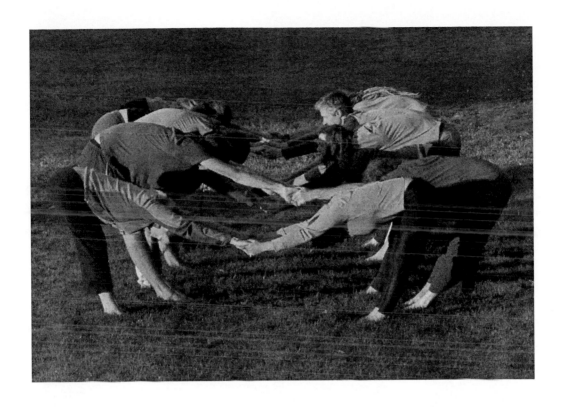

14. group child's pose (3)

DESCR: Participants start in a circle on all fours, facing the center, and slowly sink back into child's pose. Hands gently resting together with neighbor's hands.
CAUTIONS:
CALLING: "Starting on all fours, on an exhale, you can slowly sink back into child's pose. Once you're there, you can take your hands and rest them together with neighbor's hands."
NOTES:
SLANG NAMES: "Child's pose circle," "the child's garden," "childwheel."

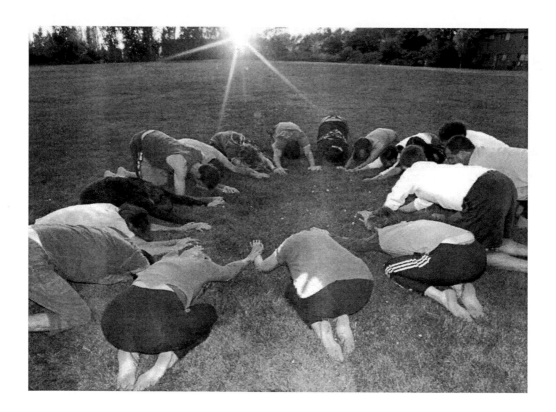

15. group ear massage (2)

DESCR: Participants sit or stand in a circle, facing the center. Hands reach up to find the earlobes of neighbors on either side.
CAUTIONS:
CALLING: "Gently, mindfully, ever so carefully, reach to find the earlobes of your neighbors on either side. And just give them a little loving ear massage."
NOTES:
VARIATIONS: Gently stretch both the ear and the neck by breathing all the heads from one side to the other.
SLANG NAMES: "Eara aura connection exercise," "I get this earie feeling we're neighbors," "the earacle speaks," "the earacles of love."

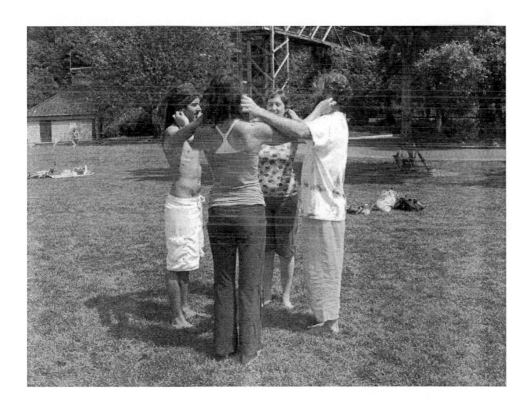

16. standing prayer hands heart circle (1)

DESCR: Participants stand in a circle, facing the center. Hands to heart center.
CAUTIONS:
CALLING: "Feet together, hands to heart center. Breathing here. Inhale, open palms to neighbors' palms. Exhale, hands to heart center. Inhale, open palms to neighbors' palms. Exhale, hands to heart center. One more time. And give a bow to the group. Namaste."
NOTES:

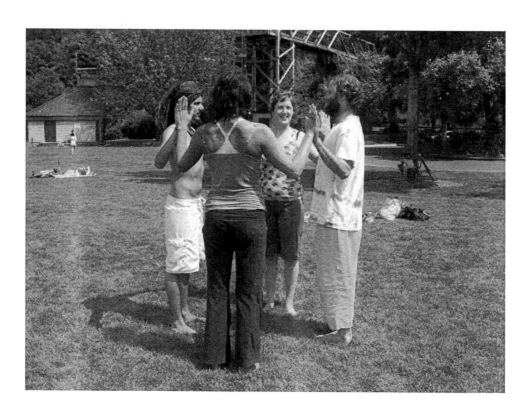

17. group spiral shavasana circle (3)

DESCR: Participants lay in a spiral circle, with head on neighbor's stomach.
CAUTIONS:
CALLING: "You're going to lay with your head on your neighbor's stomach. Heads towards the middle, feet towards the outside. All the inside hands together in the middle. Outside hand gently rests on the top of the head or crown chakra of the person in front of you. We're going to OM together 3 times. Ready? Take a big breath in... OMMMM. [pause...] OMMMM. [pause...] OMMMM. [rest in silence for a while...] And then, you can slowly bend your knees, placing your feet on the ground. Gently roll back up, and spin around so you're seated facing the center of the circle."
NOTES:
VARIATIONS: Thai massage on the feet and legs. Take a nap. Serve tea to people when they sit up.

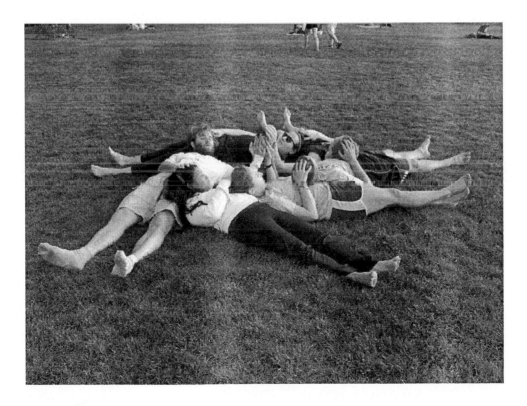

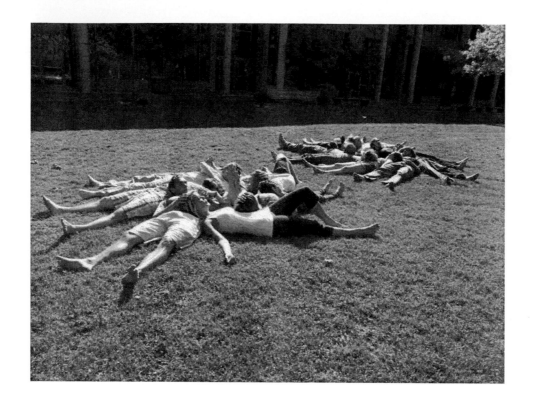

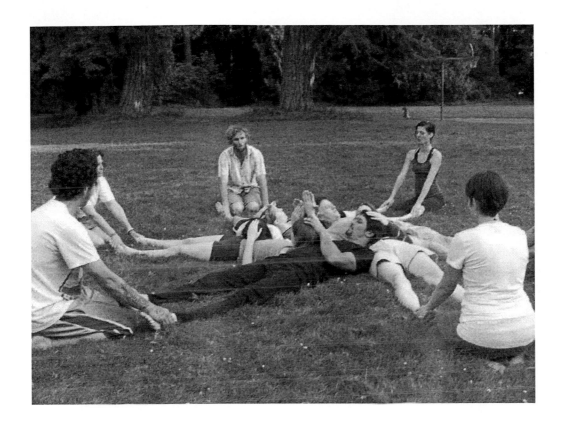

18. seated prayer hands heart circle (1)

DESCR: Participants sit in a circle, facing the center, knees touching or slightly apart.
CAUTIONS:
CALLING: "Bringing hands to heart center. Breathing here. Inhale, open palms to find neighbors' palms. Exhale, back to heart center. Inhale, open palms to find neighbors' palms. Exhale, back to heart center. And one more time. And give a bow to the group. Namaste."
NOTES:
VARIATIONS: Cross-legged, kneeling, lotus, various versions of seated.
Group hand mudras. For example, sit with first finger and thumb connected, making a small ring. Link this ring together with the rings of your neighbors on either side, making a large hoop of little ring connections.

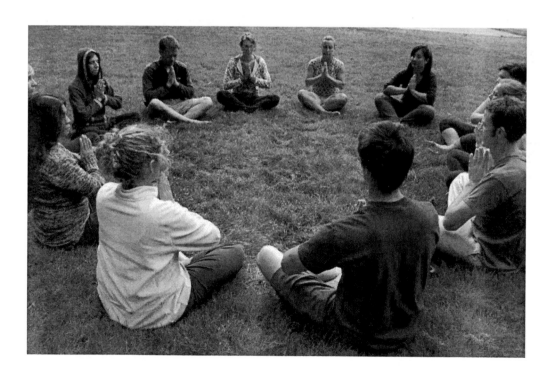

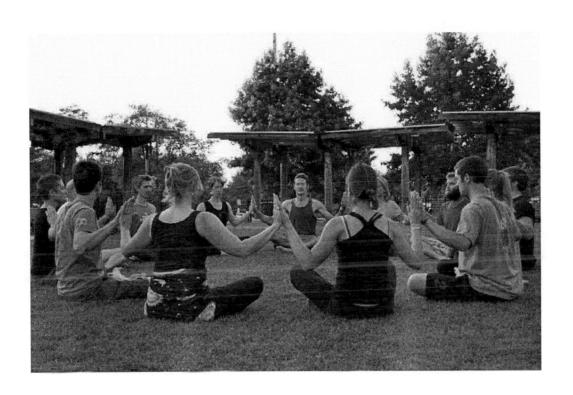

Intermediate (Levels 4-6)

Intermediate poses allow for a greater level of trust, communication, connection, skill, intention, and complexity. They are well-suited for the middle portion of a community yoga practice. There is often partial weight-sharing and support between participants. The yoga poses themselves may require a greater degree of skill, strength, flexibility, or balance.

19. hamstring square (4)

DESCR: Participants sit in a square, feet out wide. Feet to neighbors' feet.
CAUTIONS:
CALLING: "Inhale, lengthen your spine, hands up high. Exhale, folding forward toward your right foot, bringing your head toward your shin and your hands to your own right foot, or both your own right foot and your neighbor's left foot. Breathing here. Inhale, back up to center. Exhale, rest. Now we'll try the other side. Inhale, lengthen your spine…"
NOTES:
VARIATIONS: hamstring pair, triangle, pentagon, hexagon, etc.

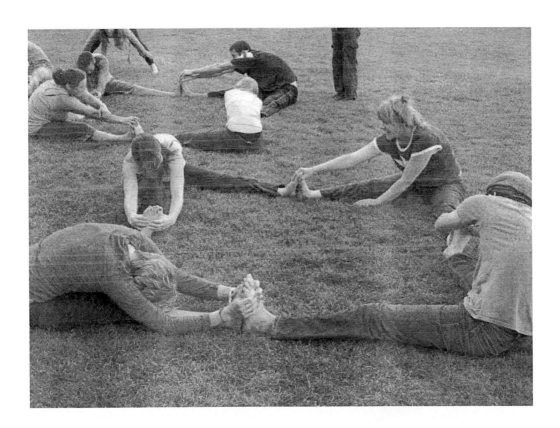

20. trivial pursuit pie carousel spin (4)

DESCR: Participants sit in a circle, backs to the center, hips to hips, feet spread apart, legs touching or resting next to neighbor's legs.
CAUTIONS:
CALLING: "Inhale, lengthen your spine and lift your hands up to shoulder height over your legs. Exhale, everyone spin to the right, bringing your hands to you and your neighbors' feet, you and your neighbors' legs, or the space in between your neighbor's legs. Breathing here. Inhale, back up to center. Exhale, rest. Now we'll try it again on the other side. Inhale, lengthen your spine..."
NOTES:
VARIATIONS: Twinkle all the hands up toward the sky.

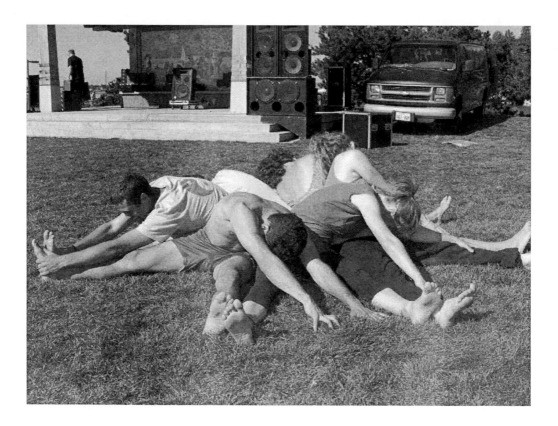

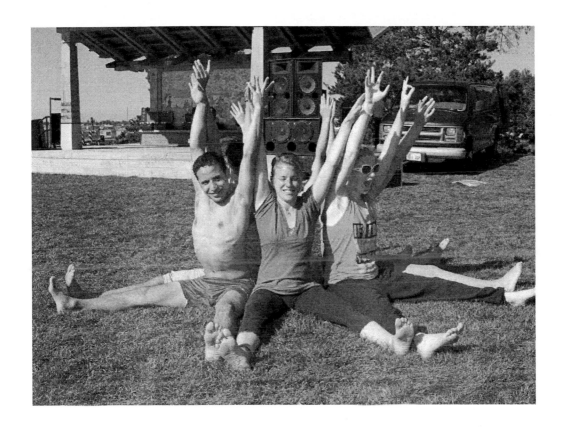

21. trivial pursuit pie straddle forward fold (5)

DESCR: Participants sit in a circle, backs to the center, hips to hips, feet spread apart, legs touching or resting next to neighbor's legs.
CAUTIONS:
CALLING: "Inhale, lengthen your spine. Exhale, forward toward your feet. Breathing here. Then see if you can bring your hands to neighbor's feet. Breathing here. Inhale, back up. Exhale, rest."
NOTES:
VARIATIONS: Back-to-back with side neighbor in pairs as you reach forward toward the feet that are next to one another in between you. Inhale, back up. Switch, same thing with other neighbor on your other side."

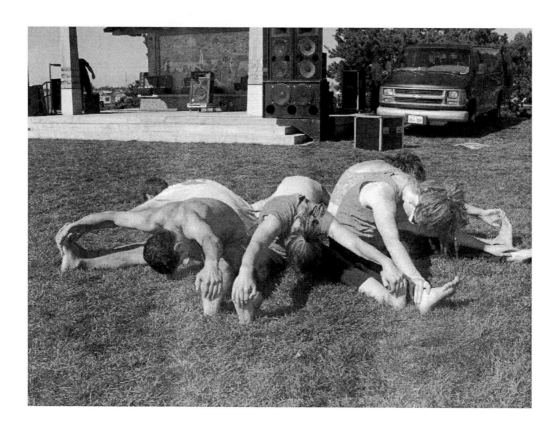

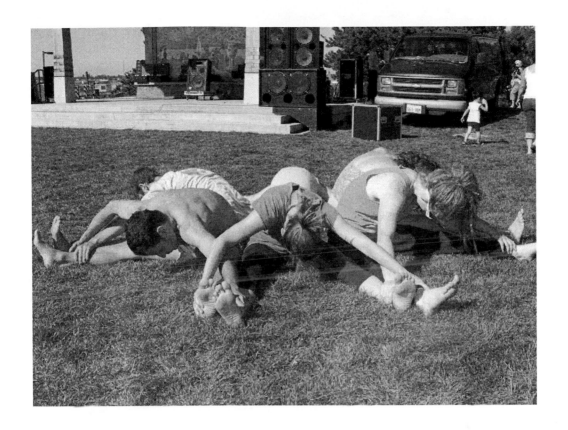

22. paper doll parade (5)

DESCR: Participants start standing in two back-to-back offset straddle lines, with sides of feet touching sides of neighbors' feet.
CAUTIONS:
CALLING: "Inhale, lengthen the spine. Exhale, folding forward to your own ankles. Breathing here. Then take your hands through your legs to the middle to grab the pair of heels (one neighbor apiece) behind you in the center of your legs. Pull yourself gently further into the stretch."
NOTES: The people at the end of the line will only have one ankle behind them between their legs. These people can take both hands to one ankle.
VARIATIONS: From the bottom, stretch to both sides, one side at a time, as in pose #52, elephant trunks, elephant ankles.
SLANG NAMES: "Paper doll ankle grab."

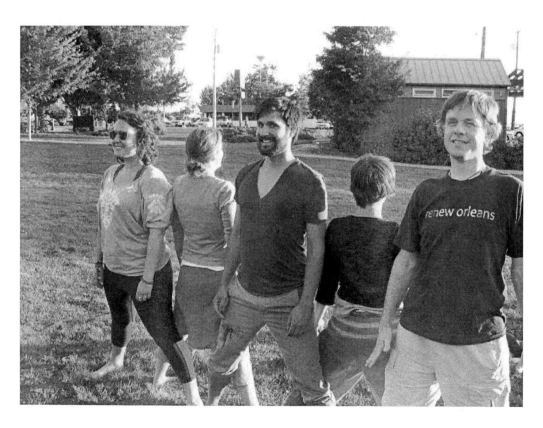

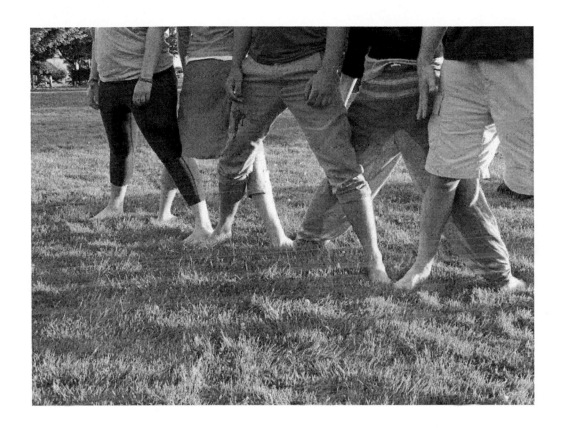

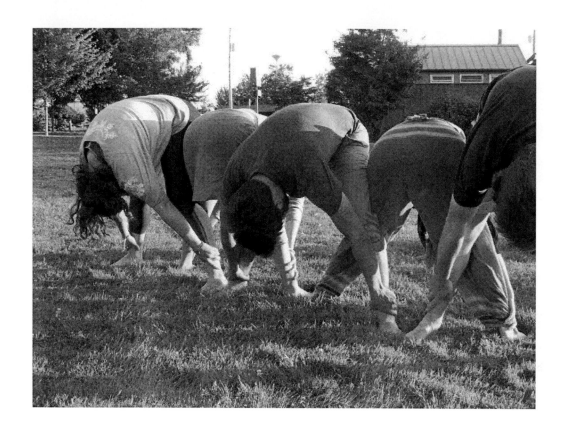

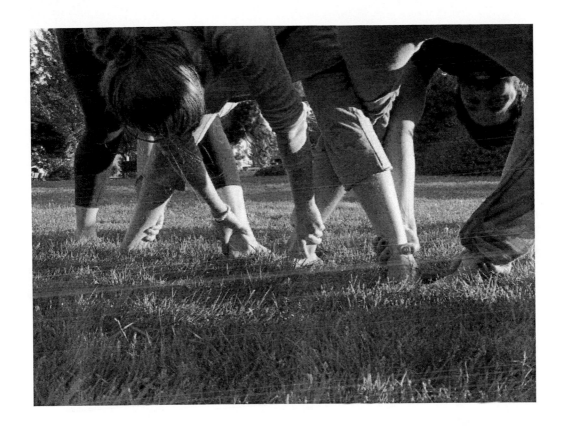

23. group tree pose (5)

DESCR: Participants stand in a circle, facing the center.
CAUTIONS:
CALLING: "Starting with hands to neighbor's shoulders, you can bring your right foot up into some version of tree pose. You could have your foot on your ankle, calf, inside of the thigh, or in lotus. Hands to heart center. Inhale, hands up the center line. Exhale here. Inhale, open your palms to the side and find your neighbors' palms. And then interlacing your fingers with your neighbors."
NOTES:
VARIATIONS: 'Trees grow tall together.' On the count of three, everyone lifts up onto the ball of the foot of the standing leg. Exhale, gently back down.
SLANG NAMES: "Friendly forest," "loving (groove) grove."

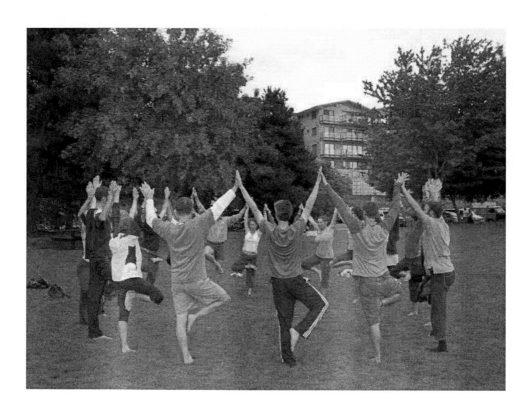

24. group spinal twist (5)

DESCR: Participants stand in a circle, facing the center.
CAUTIONS:
CALLING: "Take your right hand and fold it behind your back. Walk your feet slightly off to the right with little tiny baby steps. Now take your left hand and reach forward to find the right hand of the person in front of you (it should now be behind their back, waiting for you to grab it). Inhale, lengthen and straighten your spine, exhale, twist off to the left, looking over your left shoulder, while simultaneously feeling and maybe adding slightly to the pull of your neighbors. Inhale, back to center. Exhale, rest, letting go of the hands. And then, we'll try it again on the other side. Baby walk your feet off to the left..."
NOTES:
SLANG NAMES: "I'll twist your spine, if you twist mine," "this is spinal twist."

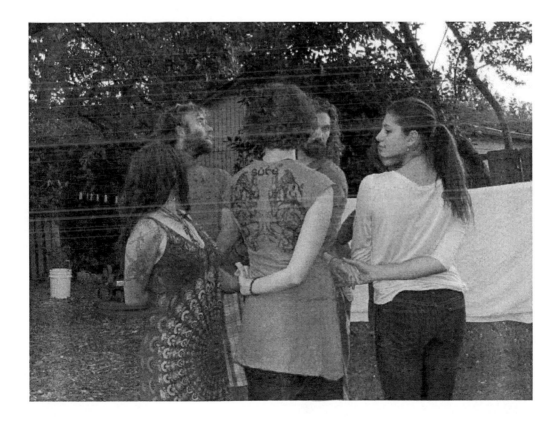

25. dancer bigtop (5)

DESCR: Participants stand in a circle, facing the center.
CAUTIONS:
CALLING: "Put your right hand into the middle, with everyone else's right hand. Take your left hand and gently grab your left foot or ankle. Take a little hop back to give yourself some space if you need it. Inhale, lengthen, straighten the spine. Exhale, hands go up in front, feet go up in back."
NOTES: Unless you're intentionally taking the hands down as an advanced variation, press up with the hands, not down.
VARIATIONS: Hop around in a circle with the hands together in the middle.

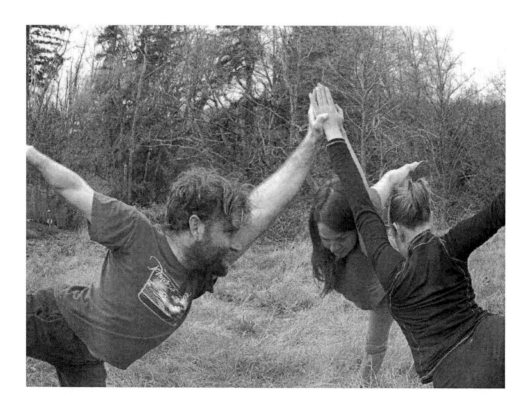

26. dancer directional circle (6)

DESCR: Participants stand in a circle, facing the center.
CAUTIONS:
CALLING: "Walk your feet gently to the right with little baby steps. Inhale, raise your right hand high and grow tall. Tall arm, tall spine, tall standing leg. Then grab your left foot with your left hand. Exhale, breathing forward, opening up into dancer pose, bringing your right hand to neighbor's ankle. Breathe a few breaths here. Inhale, back up, letting go, lifting your hand off the top. Exhale, take that hand behind you. Resting in the center. And we'll try it again on the other side. Walk your feet off to the left with little baby steps. Inhale, raise your left hand..."
NOTES:
VARIATIONS: Hand reaching forward to neighbor can gently clasp (or rest) on neighbor's foot, ankle, hip, near shoulder, or far shoulder.

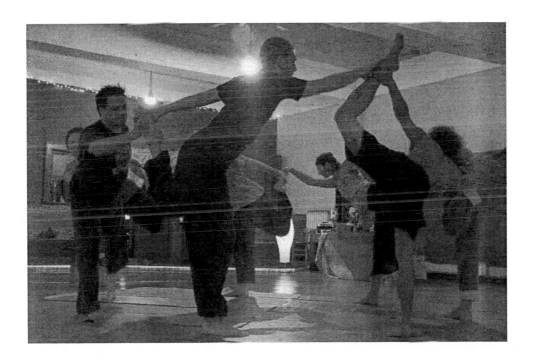

27. shared 3rd eye bow (5)

DESCR: Participants stand in a circle, facing the center, feet together, hands to heart center.
CAUTIONS:
CALLING: "Starting with the feet together, hands together at heart center, give a bow to the group. Inhale, hands up to your third eye. Breathing here. Give a bow, and back up. Inhale, open palms to the forehead or third eye of your neighbors on either side, making a shared set of prayer hands together with the hand of your 'second neighbor' on either side (the person 2 people around the circle from you). With these shared prayer hands in front of the third eye of the person right next to you on either side, give a bow."
NOTES:
VARIATIONS: Keeping palms together with both your second neighbors, breathe the hands back and forth between the circle's center and everyone's third eyes.
SLANG NAMES: "The heart of sharkness," "shared prayer shark fins," "the heart charkra salute," "getting in touch with your 3rd eye chakra," "chakra khan convention."

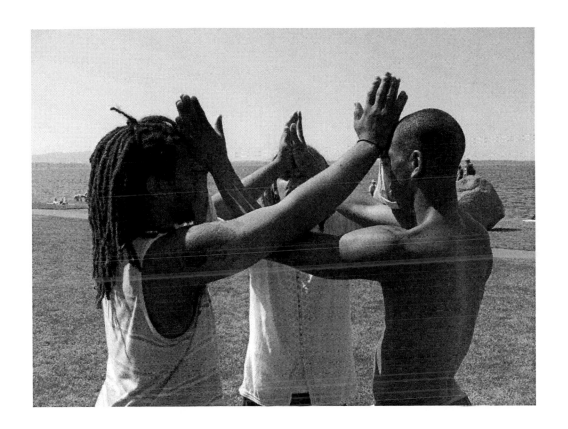

28. prayer hand flower (5)

DESCR: Participants stand in a circle, facing the center, feet together, hands to heart center.
CAUTIONS:
CALLING: "Inhale, prayer hands up to your own 3rd eye. Exhale, rest. Inhale, hands open to neighbors' 3rd eyes. Breathing here. Then, with hands at neighbor's third eyes, staying connected with the palms you're already connected with, bring the hands together into the middle, at heart level. Step back slightly to straighten the arms. Now slowly rotate your wrists up and down so the fingertips point down to the earth and back up towards the sky, making a shared prayer hand flower in the middle. Repeat 3 times. Then, let go of the shared prayer hands, and find your immediate neighbors' hands and sweep down, behind, and up and around, back to the top, back to your own palms together, slowly back down the centerline to your own heart. Give a bow to the group."
NOTES:

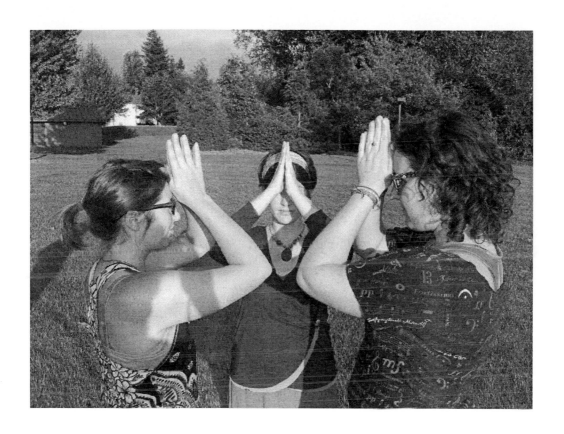

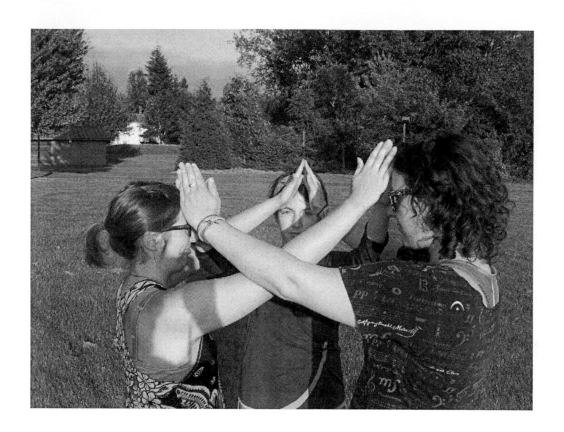

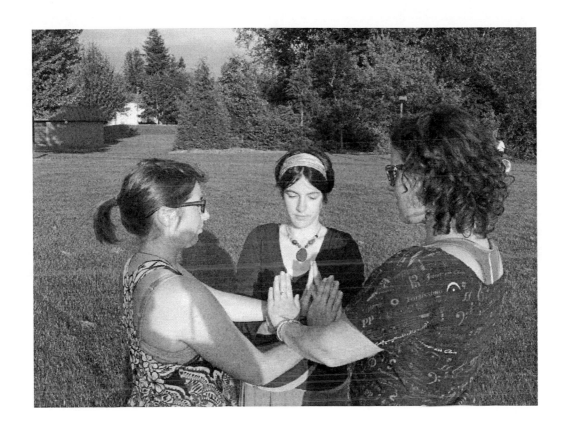

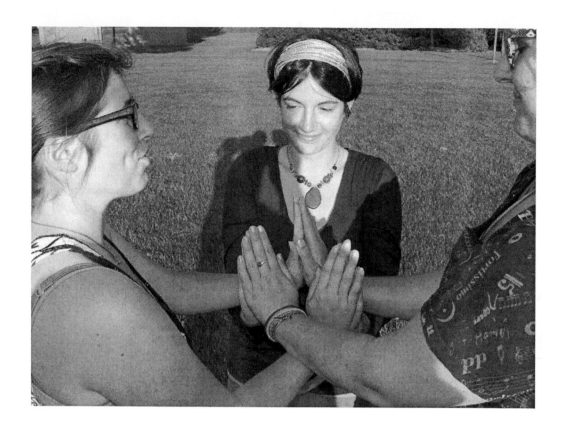

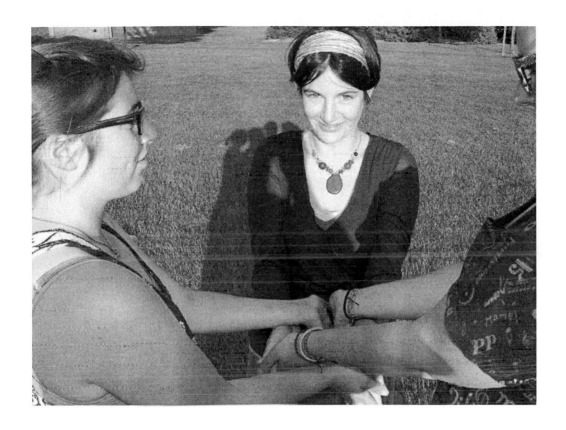

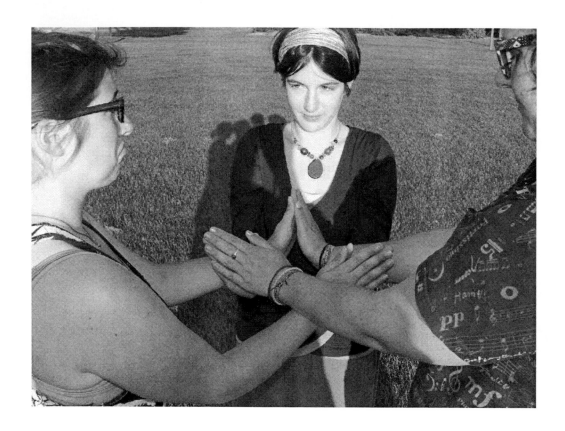

29. sunflower backbend (6)

DESCR: Participants stand in a circle, arms crossed in front. Find neighbor's hands, everyone lean and arch back into a backbend circle.
CAUTIONS: Be mindful of your neighbors. Don't pull the circle out of shape or bend way further than your neighbors are comfortable with. Don't lean to one side or the other. Stay centered.
CALLING: "Cross your arms. Find neighbor's hands. Step in a little closer. On three we're all going to lean back into a back bend together, curling the spine backwards. Ready? One, two, three... Exhale, back. [pause...] Inhale, back up to center. Cross your arms the other way, and we'll try it again..."
NOTES:
SLANG NAMES: "group backbend flower."

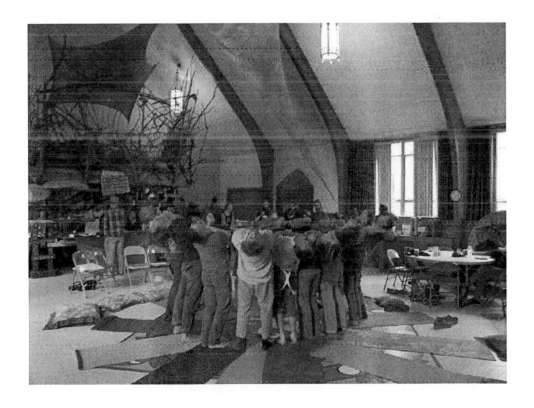

30. ski-jumper (6)

DESCR: Participants start in one or more long lines, facing one another. One person turns around, back to their partner.
CAUTIONS:
CALLING: "If you're behind, reach forward and gently grab your partner's wrists. If you're in front, exhale, slowly lean forward into a backbend, trusting your partner to hold you. Look up. Open your heart. Bring your shoulder blades together in the back. Let your hips sink forward. Inhale, back up. Exhale, rest. And we'll switch. Everyone turn around, and here we go…"
NOTES:

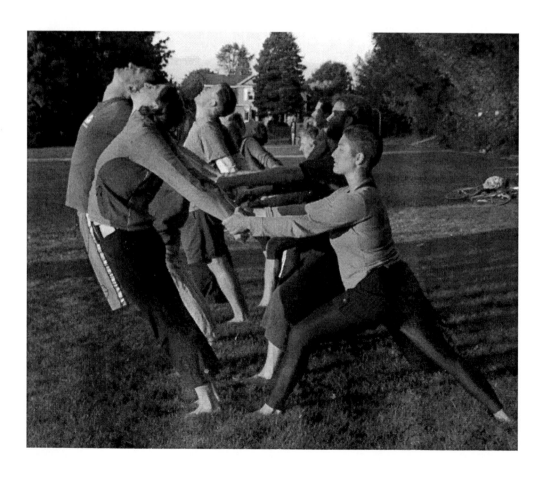

31. partner boat splits (6)

DESCR: Participants sit in facing pairs, in one or more long lines. Feet to partner's feet, with all the feet in one long line down the middle.

CAUTIONS:

CALLING: "Bend your knees, scoot forward a bit. Find neighbor's hands. Lift the feet by straightening the legs, one pair of legs at a time. Once you're up, in alternating pairs down the group line, see if you can bring your arms to the inside and take your feet out to the outside, spreading them apart, but with your feet still up in the air. And then switch, the other half of the pairs go. And switch… And then gently coming back down."

NOTES: If there is a lot of space between the pairs, all the pairs can take the feet out wide at the same time.

VARIATIONS: If partner boat is relatively easy and comfortable, participants can reach forward to grab their own (or partner's) ankles. With a straight spine, fold forward, bringing forehead toward shins.

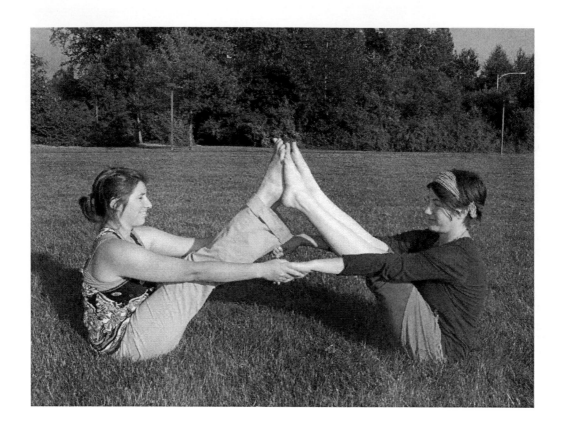

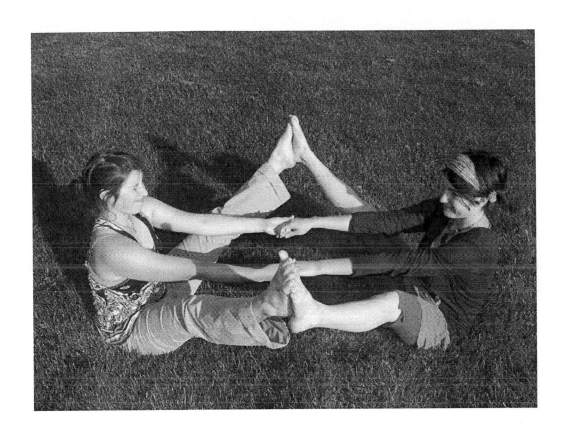

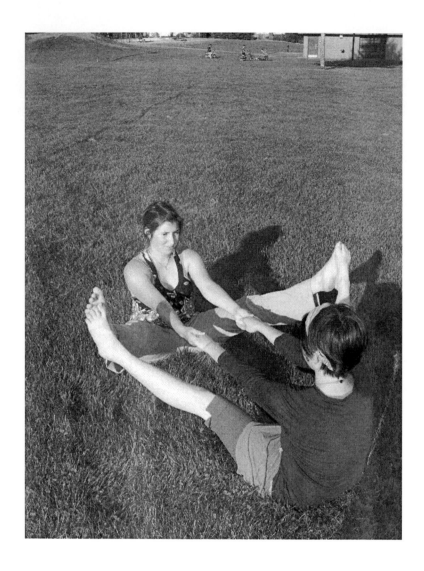

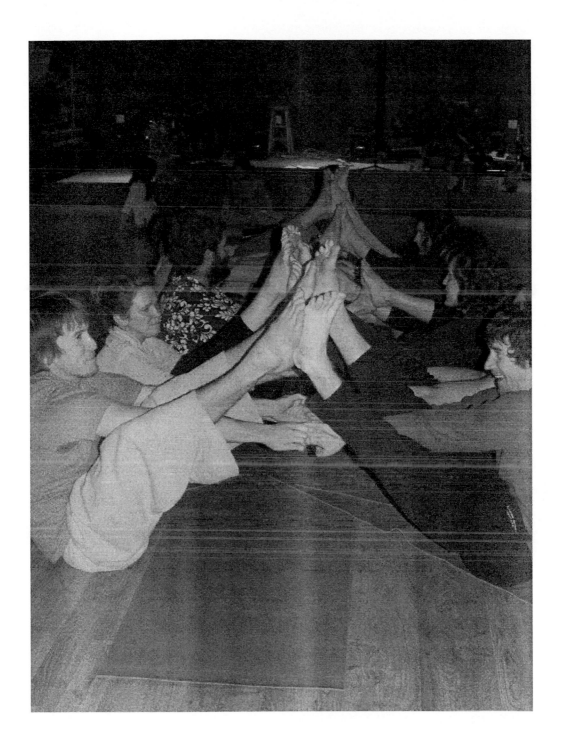

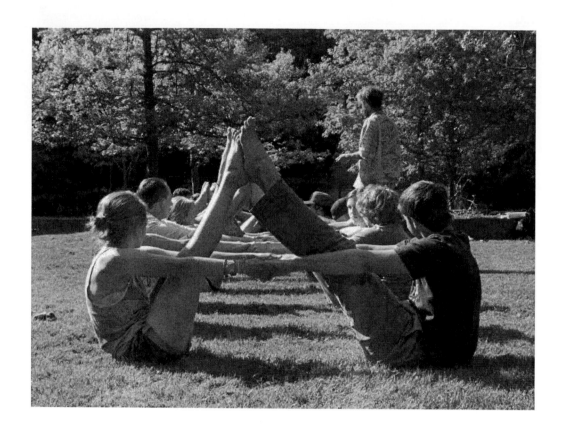

32. 3-8 person boat (6)

DESCR: Participants sit in small groups, with their feet together in the middle.
CAUTIONS:
CALLING: "Bending your knees and scooting forward a little bit, finding neighbor's hands on either side, then lifting the feet up by straightening the legs one pair at a time. Breathing here. Inhale, lengthen the spine. Exhale, lean to the right. Inhale, back to center. Exhale, rest. Inhale, lengthen the spine. Exhale, lean to the left. Inhale, back to center. Exhale, rest."
NOTES: With 4 people, it is sometimes nice to have two people who are directly opposite one another go up first, pressing the soles of their feet together, and then have the second pair go up next, bracing against the ankles of the first pair.
VARIATIONS: Grab ahold of the ankle, near foot of neighbors on either side, far foot of neighbors on either side, or neighbor directly opposite's feet.

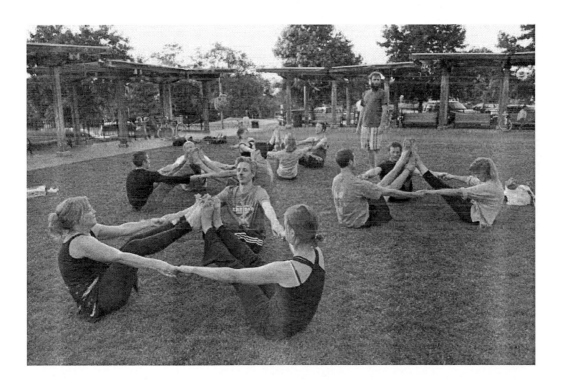

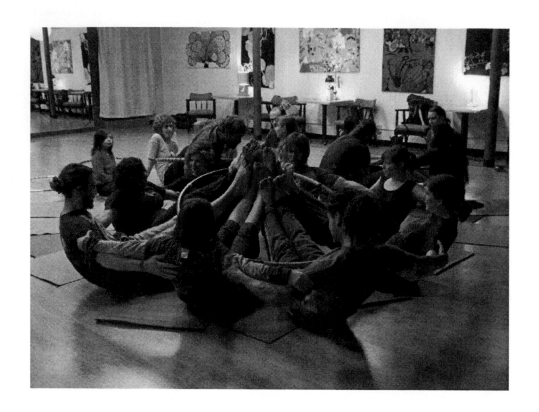

33. sidestretch paper foldouts (6)

DESCR: Participants sit in groups of 3 or 4, legs out wide, feet to neighbors' feet.
NOTES:
CALLING: "Inhale, lengthen your spine. Exhale, breathing forward with your arms crossed to find neighbor's hands. Inhale, open as a pair, stretching open the sides, pulling the 3rd person forward (if there are 3 people in the shape) or gently tugging against the other pair (if there are 4 people in the shape). Exhale, back to center. Rotate."
CAUTIONS: Don't strain your hamstrings just to reach neighbor's hands. Overlap the feet with your neighbors or bend the knees or both.
VARIATIONS: Depending on how many people are in the shape, one or two pairs can fold out at the same time.
SLANG NAMES: "Armigami."

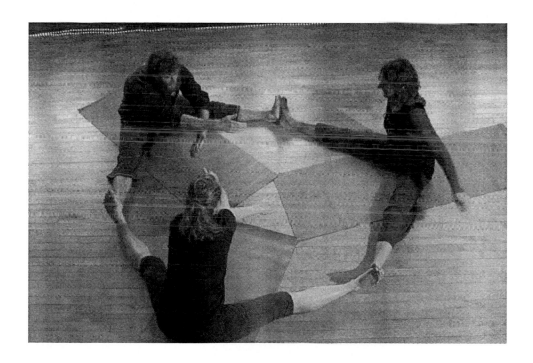

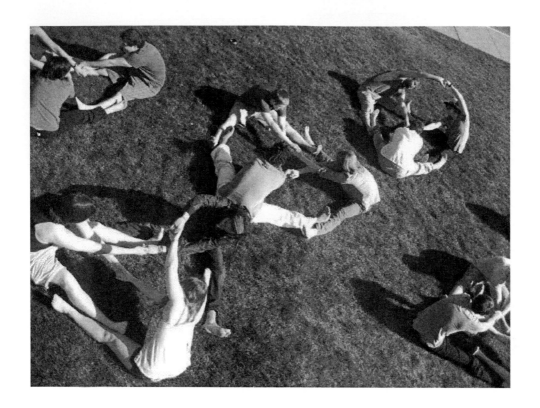

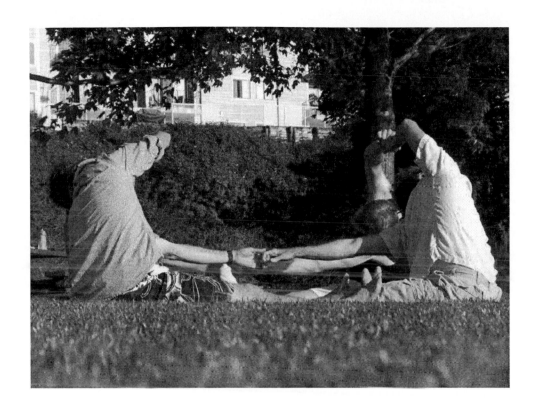

34. pinwheel (5)

DESCR: Participants sit with one foot in the middle of a circle, the opposite knee bent, with opposite foot tucked in to the inside of the thigh.
CAUTIONS:
CALLING: "Bring your right foot into the middle. Rest your foot against your neighbor's leg, in between the ankle and the calf. Take your right hand one person to the left and grab ahold of that person's foot. Inhale your left arm open behind you. Exhale back toward the center, stack everyone's hands together in a pile. Inhale open. Exhale to center. One more time. Inhale, open. Exhale, this time bring your left hand to the left, finding the left wrist of the person to your left. Gently grab ahold of their wrist. Breathing here. Inhale open, letting go, lifting the hand up. Exhale, taking the arm behind you, resting the left forearm on the ground. Right arm reaches over the top away from the circle. If you're really feeling it, raise the hips. Then lower back down. Sweep the arm to the middle. Switch the legs and we'll try the other side..."
NOTES:
VARIATIONS: After breathing forward three times, with hands on wrists and everyone breathing forward, you can try adjusting the hands slightly to interlace fingers on both hands with the second neighbor around.

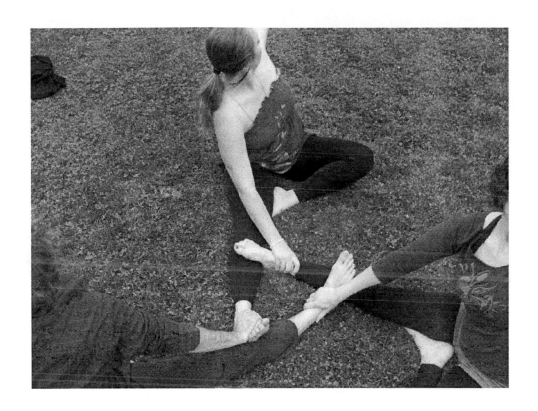

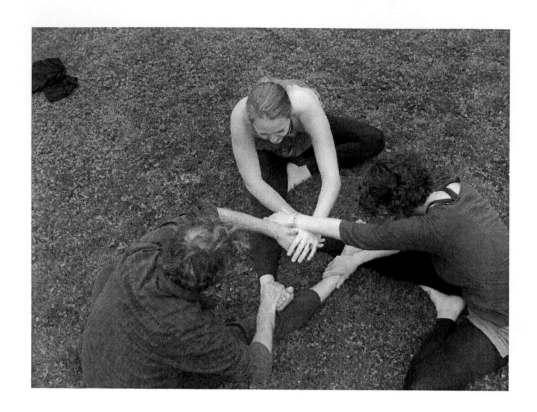

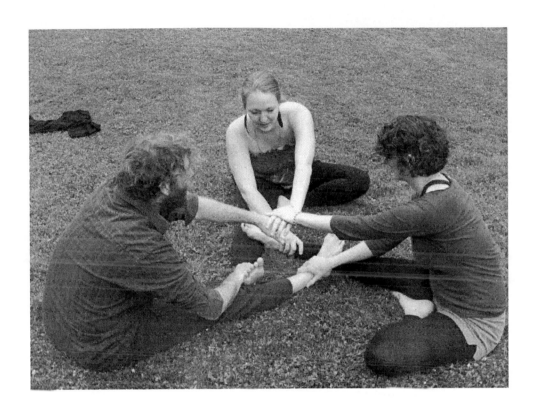

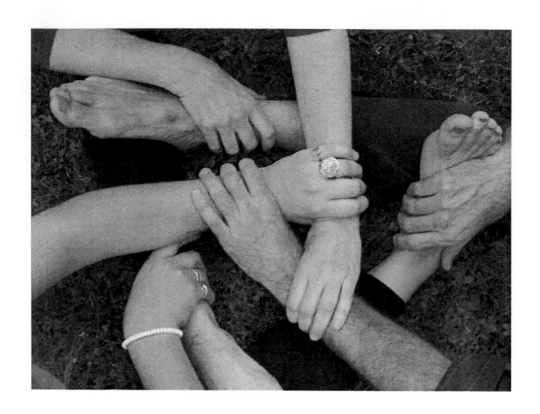

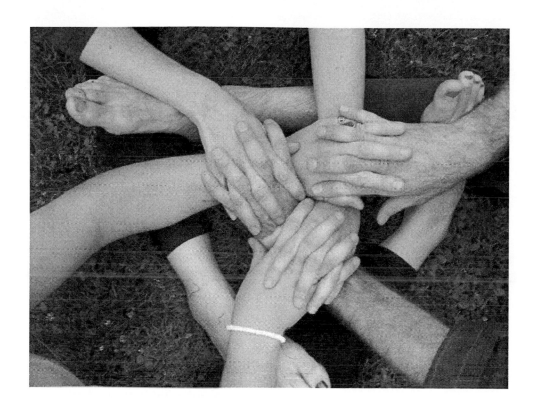

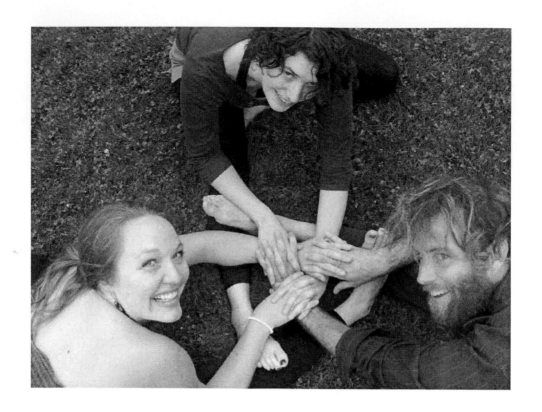

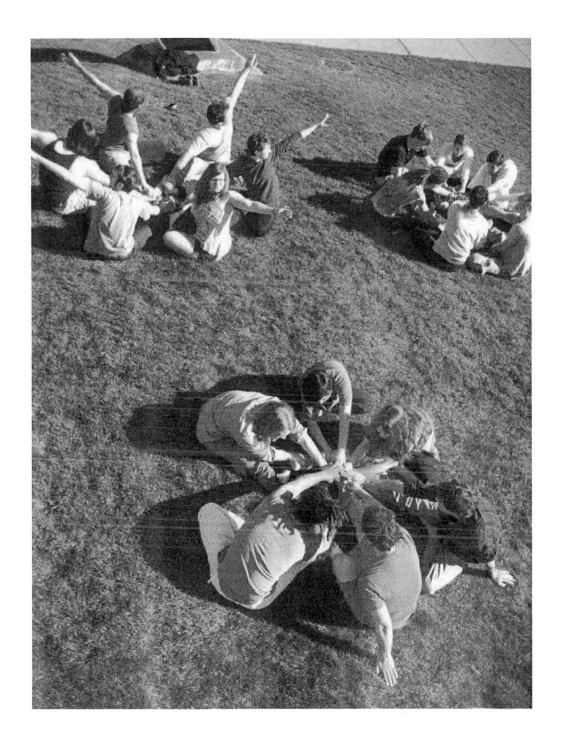

35. ship at sea (5)

DESCR: Participants sit in one or more long lines, in a straddle, feet-to-feet with the person in front of them, back to back with the person behind them.
CAUTIONS:
CALLING: "Inhale, lengthen your spine. Exhale, everyone fold toward the North (South, West, East, etc.). Inhale, back to center. Exhale, rest. Inhale, lengthen your spine. Exhale, everyone fold toward the South (North, East, West, etc.). If you're folding forward, you can reach forward to your own shins, ankles, or feet. Or you can reach for your neighbor's shins, ankles, or feet. If you're leaning backwards, you can rest your back on the person behind you and let your arms sweep up overhead. If you're on the end of the group line and you're leaning backwards out into empty space, you can reach your arms forward to find the hands or wrists of the person in front of you."
NOTES:
SLANG NAMES: "Poor folks' roller coaster," "ship-at-sea straddles."
RELATED POSES: See also, pose #59, spider.

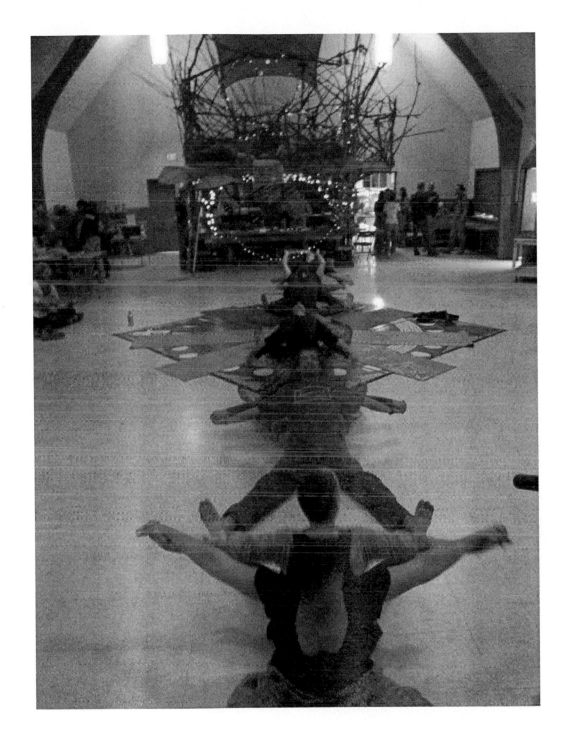

36. caterpillar east and west (6)

DESCR: Participants sit back-to-back in two lines, legs out straight in front.
CAUTIONS:
CALLING: "Now we're all going to go East [towards that tree, famous landmark, etc, over there.] So this line, facing East, exhale forward, reaching towards your feet, forehead towards the shins. This other line, facing West, inhale your hands straight up over your head and behind you, gently allowing your weight to help press the person underneath you a little further into the stretch."
NOTES:
VARIATIONS: For a deeper stretch for those underneath, people in the line raising their hands up overhead, can bend their knees, place their feet on the ground, and press up into a version of tabletop with their hands still in the air behind them.

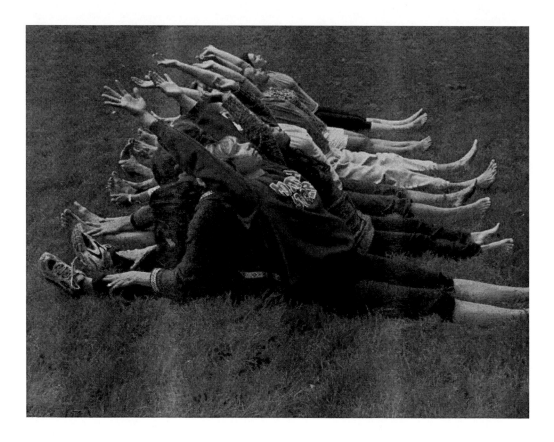

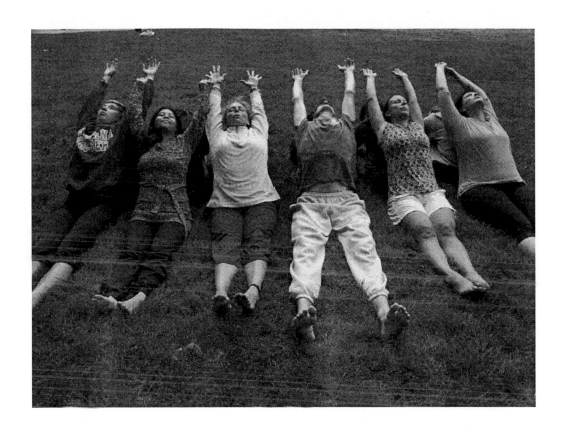

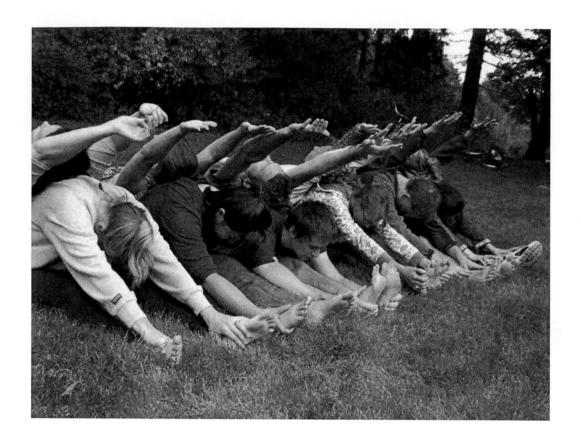

37-41. CLASSIC SEQUENCE #2: butterflies (6)

37. butterfly twist line (6)

DESCR: Participants sit back-to-back in two lines, knees touching or almost touching neighbors' knees.
CAUTIONS:
CALLING: "Inhale, lengthen and straighten your spine. Exhale, twist to your own right, taking your right hand to neighbor's left knee behind you. Inhale, back to center. Exhale, rest. And now we'll try it again on the other side..."
NOTES:
VARIATIONS: 'The Extra Twist-a-pede.' Reach across a little further to the knee of the person behind you at a diagonal. In mosaic, reach behind and interlace fingers with the person two places behind you and one place to the side.
SLANG NAMES: "Twist-a-pede."

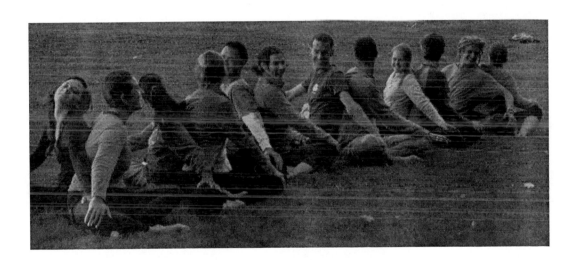

38. butterfly neck rest (6)

DESCR: Participants sit with their spines back-to-back, cross-legged, in baddha konasana, or in lotus.
CAUTIONS:
CALLING: "Inhale, take your head and neck back to the right, resting on partner's shoulder, looking up. Exhale, back to center. Now the other side. Inhale, take your head and neck back to the left, resting on partner's shoulder, looking up. Exhale, back to center. Rest."
NOTES:
VARIATIONS: Hold the pose longer. Breathe.
SLANG NAMES: "The neck nuzzler," "partner stargazer."

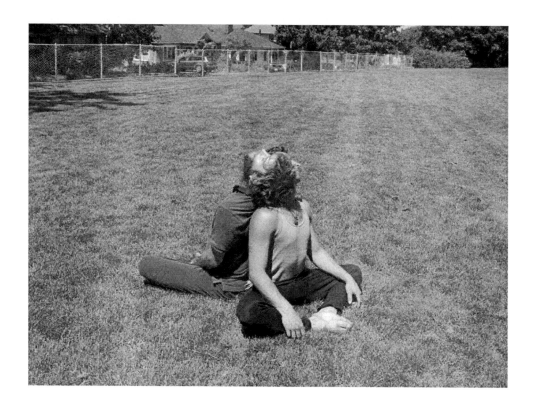

39. butterfly breathing (5)

DESCR: Participants sit back-to-back, cross-legged, in baddha konasana, or in lotus.
CAUTIONS: Nice and gentle the first time up.
CALLING: "You're going to sit back-to-back with your partner, making sure your spines are nice and straight. Now take your hands out to the sides and find your partner's hands. Interlace your fingers with that person, and then, nice and slowly on the first one, inhale up together, and then exhale back down together, all the way to the floor. Inhale up... exhale down... Inhale up... exhale down... rest."
NOTES: If one person's arms are noticeably longer than their partner's arms, the person with shorter arms can have their hands on the wrists or forearms of the person with longer arms.
VARIATIONS: If sitting cross-legged or in lotus is difficult, participants may sit with the legs out straight. If several pairs line up together laterally, 2 pairs at a time can reach toward one another and find 4 hands together, connecting with the neighboring pair. With hands to neighbors' shoulders, breathing forward in two long lines, foreheads toward the floor.
SLANG NAMES: "Flock of seagulls," "seated flying."

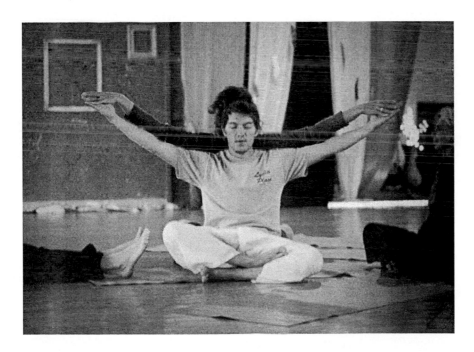

40. butterfly side-stretches (6)

DESCR: Participants sit back-to-back with a partner, cross-legged, in baddha konasana, or in lotus.

CAUTIONS: Nice and slow on the first one. Especially if one partner has tight shoulders or shorter arms.

CALLING: "Sitting back-to-back with your partner, take your hands out to the sides and find partner's hands. Interlace your fingers with your partner. Nice and slow on the first one. Inhale, up together. Exhale, fold off to one side. Bend your elbow, forearm on the ground, reach the other arm over the top and out the side. Looking up. And inhale back up to center. Exhale rest. And now the other side. Inhale, lifting up together. Exhale, folding off to the other side. Bend your elbow, forearm on the ground, reach the other arm over the top and out the side. Looking up. And inhale back up to center. Exhale rest."

NOTES: If one partner's arms are significantly longer than their partner's, the person with shorter arms can have their hands on the elbows, forearms or wrists of the person with longer arms.

VARIATIONS: Instead of all pairs breathing and folding in the same direction down the entire line, pairs can breathe towards one another to make groups of 4 people connecting hands in the middle.

SLANG NAMES: "Butterflies stretch their wings."

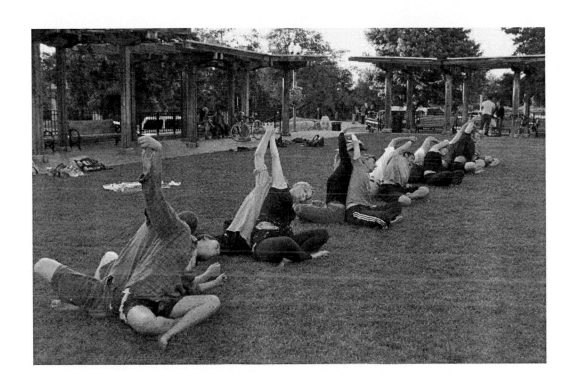

41. butterfly tabletop press (6)

DESCR: Participants sit back-to-back with a partner, cross-legged, in baddha konasana, or in lotus, in one or more long lines.
CAUTIONS: Do not support the weight of someone who is more than 25 pounds heavier than you are.
CALLING: "Sitting back-to-back with your partner, decide who's going to go first. Whoever is pressing up into tabletop, place your feet on the ground and start to lift your hips off the floor. If you're in butterfly (baddha konasana), slowly exhale forward, allowing the weight of your partner to assist you in deepening into the stretch. Breathing here. Slowly coming back up to center. Rest. Switch roles and repeat."
NOTES:
VARIATIONS: With both partners sitting back-to-back, link arms around one another's elbows and straighten the legs to stand up.

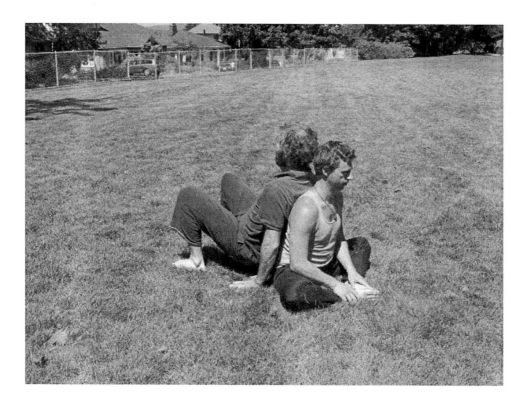

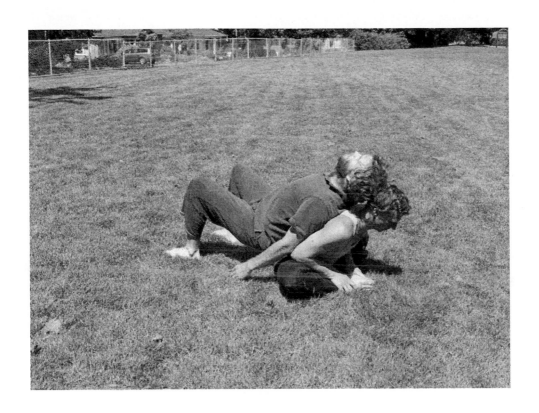

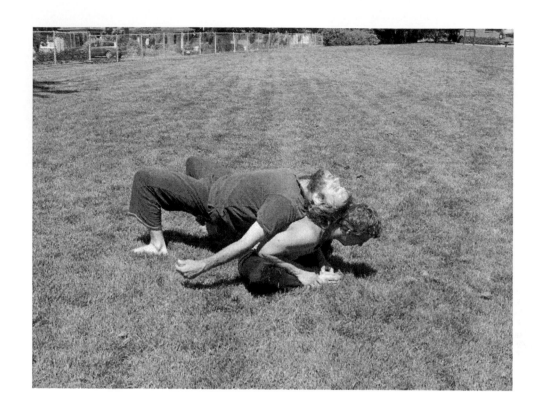

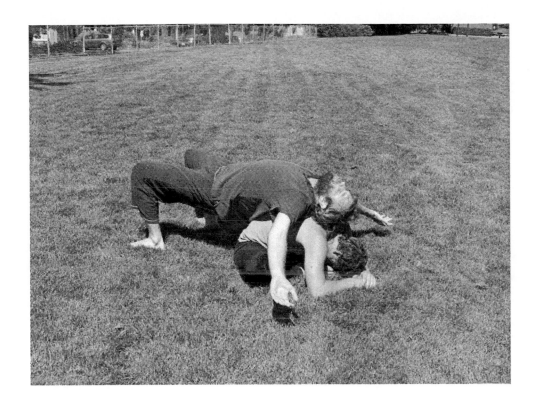

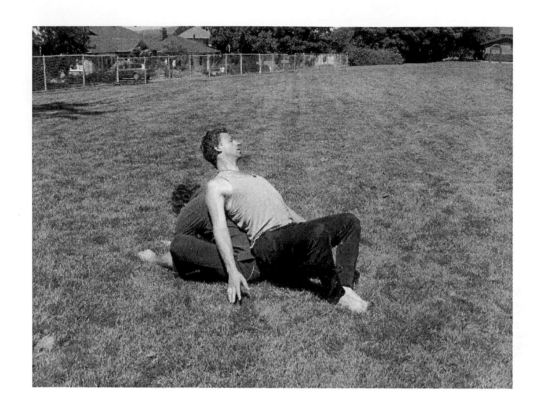

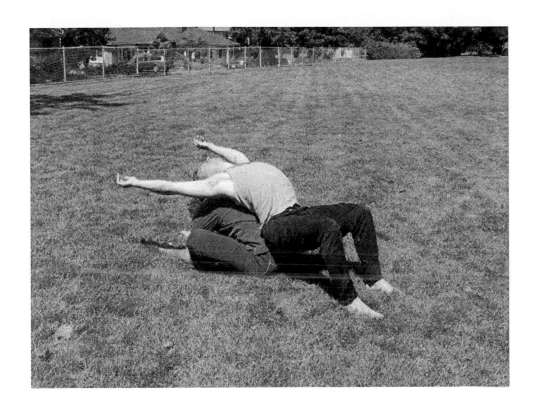

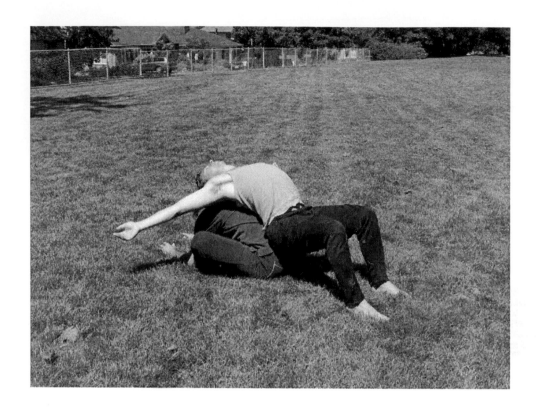

42. partner straddle see-saw line (6)

DESCR: Participants sit in a straddle, in facing pairs, in one or more long lines. Feet to partner's feet, with all the feet in one long line down the middle.
CAUTIONS: Don't strain your hamstrings just to reach partner's hands. Bend your knees if necessary to keep this safe.
CALLING: "Reaching out in front of you to find partner's hands or wrists. And then we're just gonna slowly see-saw back and forth. If you're breathing forward, it's an exhale. If you're leaning back, it's an inhale. Nice and slow. Go and ahead and give it a try."
NOTES:
VARIATIONS: Stay and hold the stretch longer. Breathe. Various grips can be used, depending on flexibility. If it is a long stretch, just the last joint of the fingers can interlock with partner. If more flexible, you can crawl up the wrist or arm.

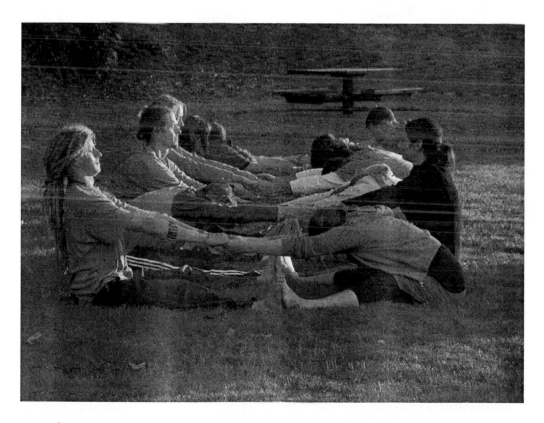

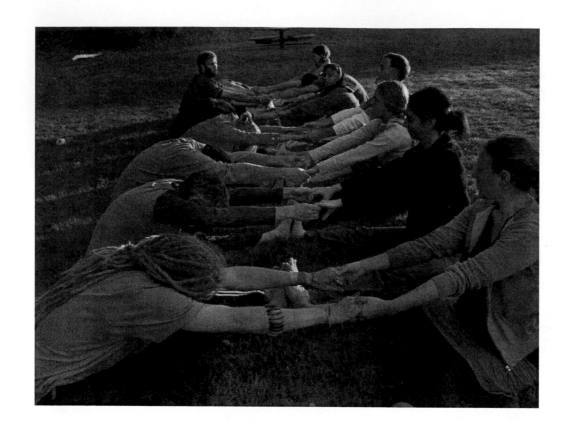

43. grass-in-the-wind (6)

DESCR: Participants sit in a straddle in facing pairs, in one or more long lines. Feet to partner's feet, with all the feet in one long line down the middle.

CAUTIONS: Don't strain your hamstrings just to reach the diagonal neighbor's hand. Bend your knees if necessary to keep this safe.

CALLING: "Okay, so we're going to come into two long lines, seated in a straddle with someone directly in front of you. Scooting slightly forward or back so all the feet line up in one big long line. Reach your right hand out in front of you to find partner's right hand or wrist. Inhale, lengthen and straighten your spine. Exhale, take your left hand over the top toward your right, finding the hand of your diagonal neighbor, or, if you're on the very end of the group shape, one or both feet. Breathing here. Inhale, back up to center and switch hands. Exhale, over to the other side. Repeat."

NOTES:

VARIATIONS: Stay and hold the stretch longer. Breathe. If the diagonal neighbor is too far to reach you can just wave to that person. Various grips can be used, depending on flexibility. If it is a long stretch, just the last joint of the fingers can interlock with partner. If more flexible, you can crawl up the wrist or arm.

RELATED POSES: See also, pose #86, grass-in-the-wind hexagon.

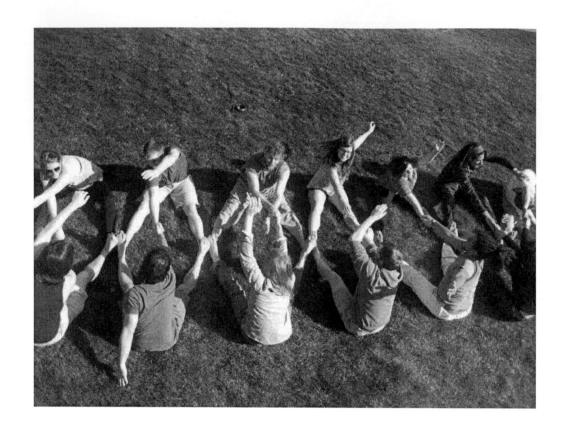

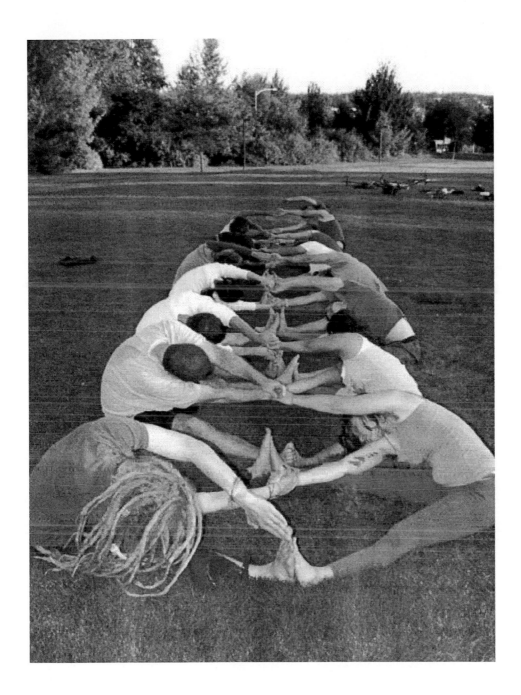

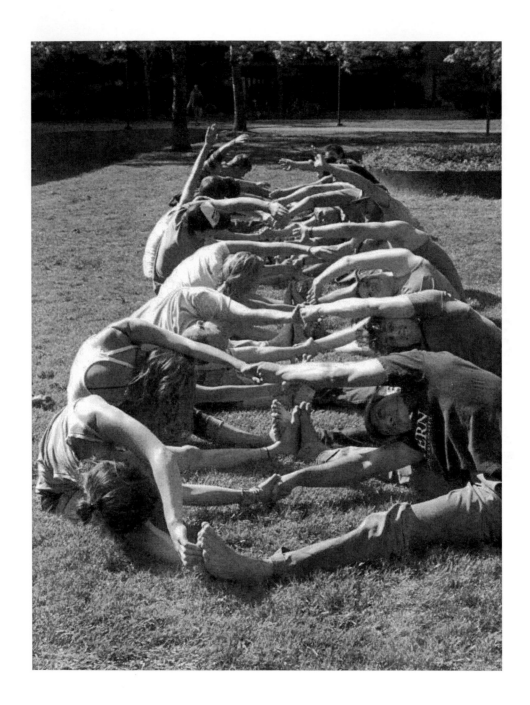

44-48. CLASSIC SEQUENCE #3: baddha konasana clover (6)

44. baddha konasana clover forward fold (6)

DESCR: Participants sit in small groups, soles of the feet together, knees folded out to the sides.
CAUTIONS: Depending on flexibility, you may want to scoot back a little so the heads don't bonk into one another when breathing forward. Or, you can stack one on top of the other, or rest on one another's shoulders if you like.
CALLING: "Inhale, lengthen the spine. Exhale, fold forward, bringing your hands to the far sides of your neighbors' feet."
NOTES:
VARIATIONS: Grab ahold of the ankle, heel, shin, calf, near foot, or far foot, of neighbors on either side, or neighbor directly opposite. Those who are particularly flexible can give a 3rd eye blessing to their neighbors, by bringing their forehead to rest on neighbor's wrists.

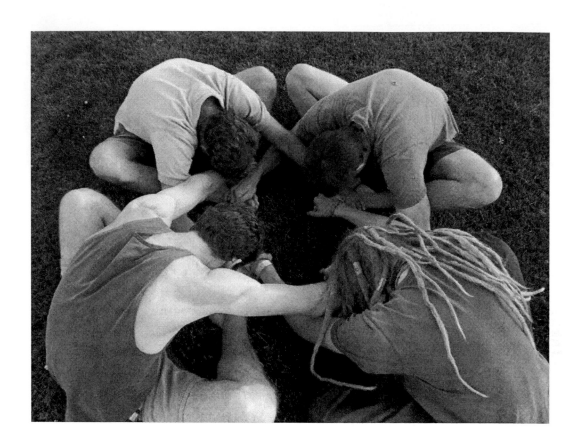

45. baddha konasana clover hands to knees (5)

DESCR: Participants sit in small groups, soles of the feet together, knees folded out to the sides.
CAUTIONS:
CALLING: "Inhale, lengthen and straighten your spine, resting hands gently on neighbor's knees, just feeling the energy of the group. Breathing here."
NOTES: Tall, straight spine.

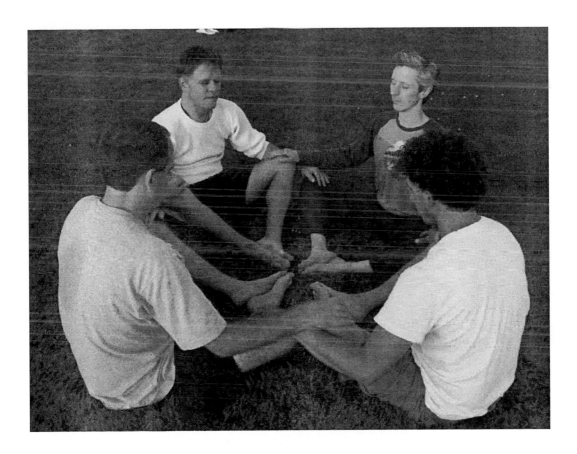

46. baddha konasana clover huddle (6)

DESCR: Participants sit in small groups, soles of the feet together, knees folded out to the sides.
CAUTIONS:
CALLING: "Inhale, lengthen and straighten your spine. Exhale, breathing forward, bringing hands to neighbors' shoulders, or to the backs of the hearts. Fingers interlaced, or hands resting on top of one another. Breathing together here."
NOTES:

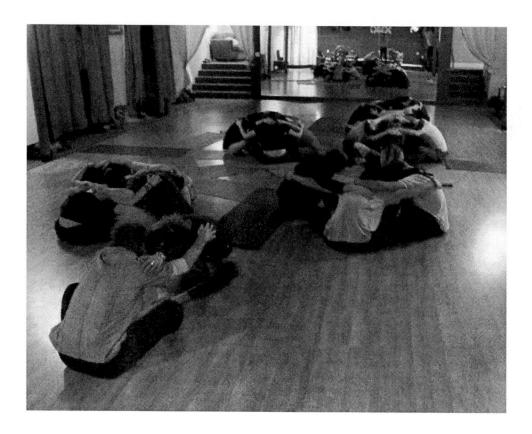

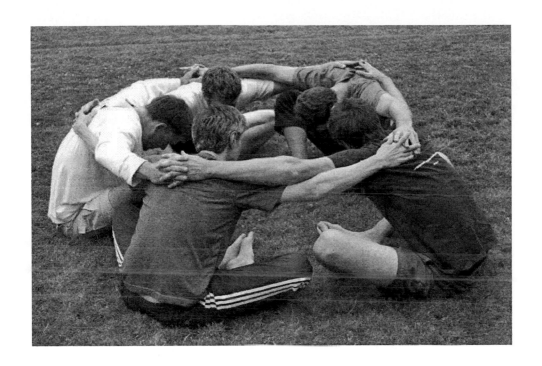

47. baddha konasana clover stir the pot (5)

DESCR: Participants sit in small groups, soles of the feet together, knees folded out to the sides.
CAUTIONS:
CALLING: "Bring your right fingertips into the center, curl them together with the rest of your group. Bring your left fingertips together in the center underneath your right hand, curl them together with the rest of your group. Now swirl the arms around together. Pause. Switch directions, swirling around the other way. Rest."
NOTES:
VARIATIONS: One hand up, one hand down, bend the elbow of the arm on bottom, and lean in towards the center. Switch, repeat.
SLANG NAMES: "Hip stew."

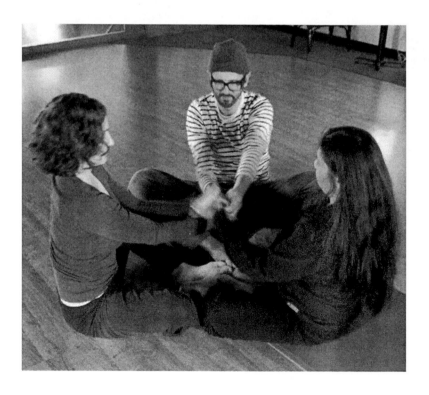

48. baddha konasana clover eggbeaters (5)

DESCR: Participants sit in small groups, soles of the feet together, knees folded out to the sides.
CAUTIONS:
CALLING: "Bring your right fingertips into the center, curl them together with the rest of your group. Bring your left fingertips together in the center underneath your right hand, curl them together with the rest of your group. Now swirl the arms around together in offset orbits. Pause. Switch directions, swirling around the other way. Rest."
NOTES:

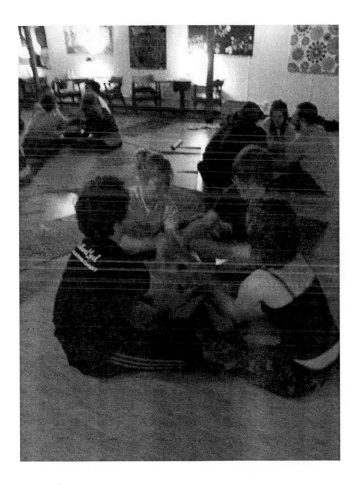

49. ballet leg lifts (6)

DESCR: Participants stand in a circle, facing the center, hands to neighbors' shoulders.
CAUTIONS:
CALLING: "On three, we're all going to lift our right legs up and out to the side at the same time. Ready? One, two, three... Lift. And again. Lift. And again. Lift. Rest. Breathing here. And now the other side..."
NOTES:
SLANG NAMES: "Pleasant ballet stretch," "neurotic ballet," "neurotic ballet warm-up."

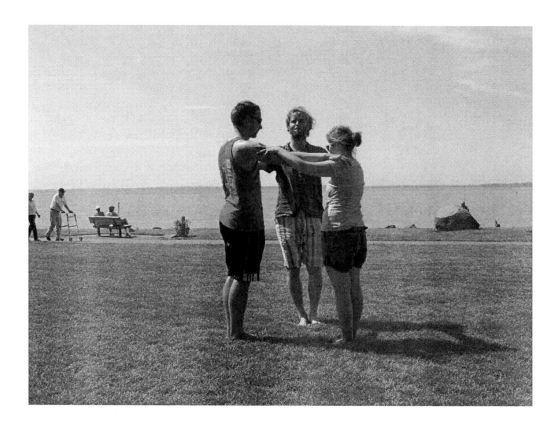

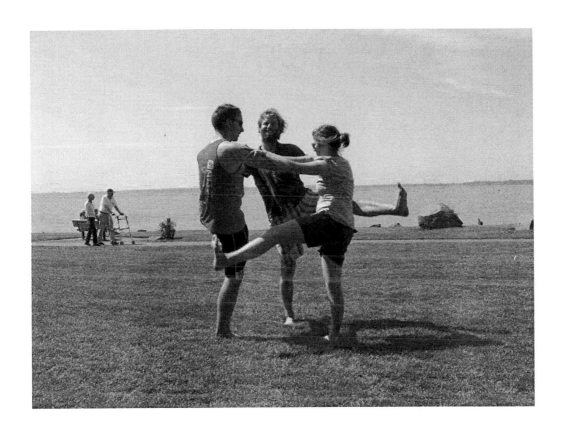

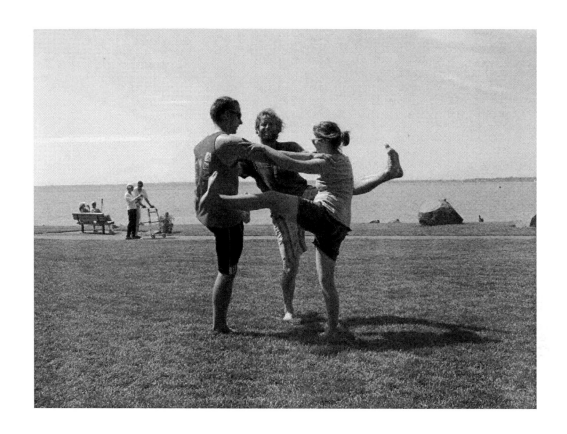

50. eagle arms line (6)

DESCR: Participants stand in a line. Cross arms as in eagle pose.
CAUTIONS:
CALLING: "Take the elbows forward and up. Exhale, fold the hands down to find neighbor's hands. Shake hands with your neighbors on either side. Inhale, back up into eagle arms. Repeat."
NOTES:
VARIATIONS: Cross legs as in eagle pose as well. While the hands are connected with neighbors' hands in one big long line, make waves with the arms across the line.

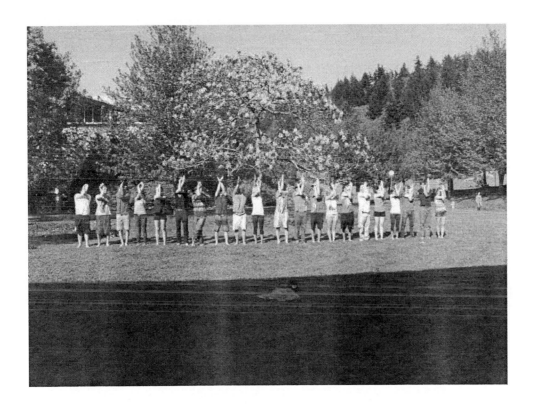

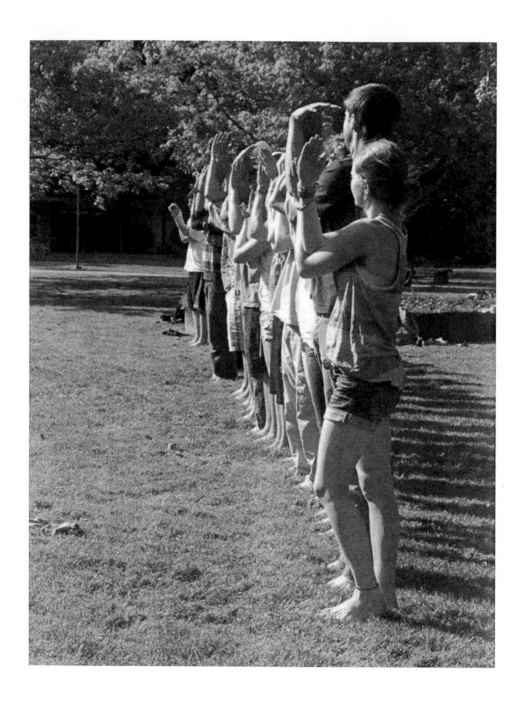

51. eagle arms cosmic spiral squawk walk in a circle (6)

DESCR: Participants stand in a circle, facing the center, in groups of 3-8 people.
CAUTIONS:
CALLING: "Cross your right arm over your left arm, as in eagle pose. Exhale, arms forward, bringing your right fingertips into the center of the circle. Curl your hand together with the rest of your group. Walk in a circle, squawking and making your best eagle noises."
NOTES:
VARIATIONS: 'Eagles perch on trees.' From eagle squawk walk, let go of the group's hands and come directly up into group tree pose.

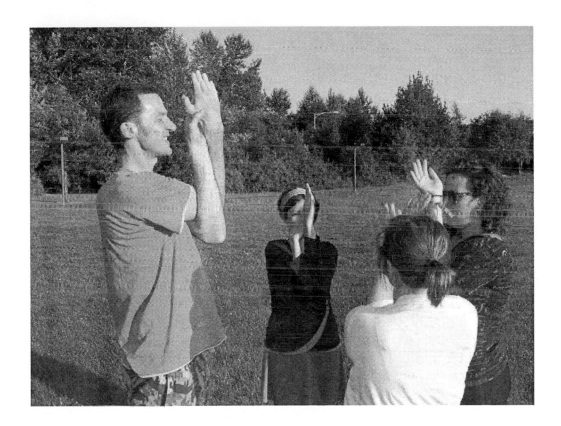

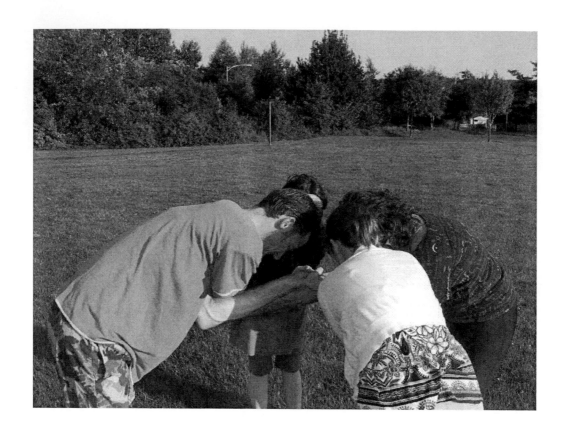

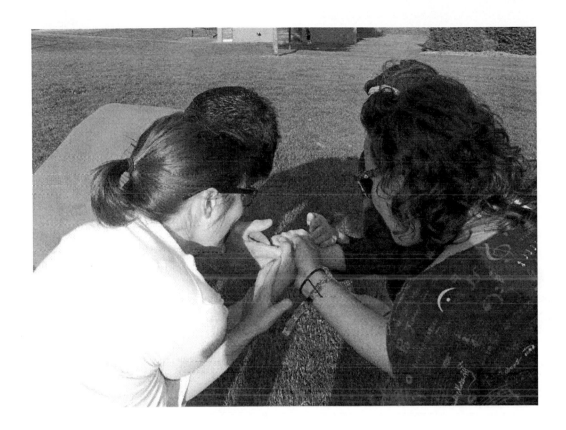

52. elephant trunks, elephant ankles (6)

DESCR: Heels next to neighbor's heels in a standing straddle, facing away from the center of the circle.
CAUTIONS:
CALLING: "Starting with your heels next to your neighbor's heels in a wide, but comfortable standing straddle, facing away from the center of the circle. Exhale, fold forward, sliding your hands down your legs to your own ankles. Inhale, slightly lift, straighten the spine. Exhale, torso to the right, your right hand to neighbor's left ankle, your left hand to your own right ankle. Breathing here. Release, back to center. Rest. Repeat on other side."
NOTES:
SLANG NAMES: "Troll-hair convention."

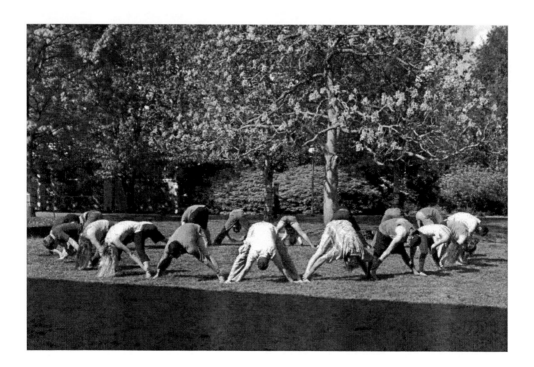

53. pigeon circle (6)

DESCR: Participants start kneeling in a circle, on all fours, facing the center. Bend one knee and bring leg forward into pigeon, other leg out long behind.
CAUTIONS:
CALLING: "Bringing hands gently to rest together with neighbor's hands. Inhale, lift, looking up or back. Exhale, folding forward into pigeon. Breathing here. Repeat 3 times."
NOTES:
VARIATIONS: Bend the knee of the back leg, grab ahold of foot or ankle. Elbow around ankle. Foot to head.
SLANG NAMES: "Central Park," "penta-pigeon," "octo-pigeon," "dodeca-pigeon," etc.
RELATED POSES: See also, pose #80, pigeon pairs.

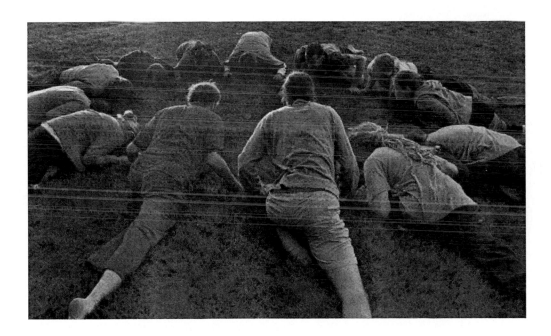

54. pigeon huddle (6)

DESCR: Participants start in pigeon circle.
CAUTIONS: Be gentle. The hands and arms do add extra weight, and they are no longer underneath you helping to support you.
CALLING: "Lifting your hands gently up to rest on neighbor's shoulders, or the backs of neighbors' hearts. Resting hands on top of the hands, or interlacing the fingers together. Breathing here."
NOTES:
SLANG NAMES: "Pigeon skydive," "pigeon earthdive," "pigeon faceplant."
RELATED POSES: See also, pose #80, pigeon pairs.

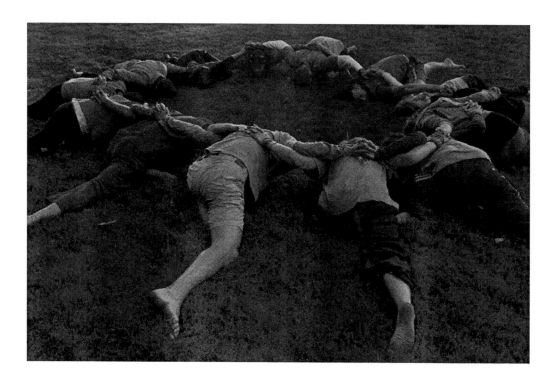

Advanced (Levels 7-9)

Advanced poses are for more flexible, experienced students of community yoga. Participants are often lifted completely off the ground, are inverted, or are sharing partial or full body weight with another person. The yoga poses themselves are often more delicate, difficult, and intricate, requiring more strength, balance or flexibility. These poses should only be practiced after thoroughly warming up with beginner and intermediate poses.

55. skydive circle (7)

DESCR: Participants stand in a circle, shoulder to shoulder, facing the center.
CAUTIONS:
CALLING: "Take your hands to neighbor's shoulders and then reach around a little further behind your neighbors' backs to what we call the second neighbors' hands. Interlace your fingers with both your second neighbors. Then lower this big long rope of the arms that we've created to the backs of the hearts. Take a few breaths here. Raise your right foot toward the center of the circle, and then swing it behind you. Give a little hop backwards. And again. And maybe one more time if need be. Now, exhale forward, head down, heel up. Breathing here several breaths. Letting go of the hands, inhale back up, walking back in. Hands to shoulders, we'll try it again on the other side..."
NOTES:
SLANG NAMES: "Skydiving without all that expensive equipment," "earthdiving."

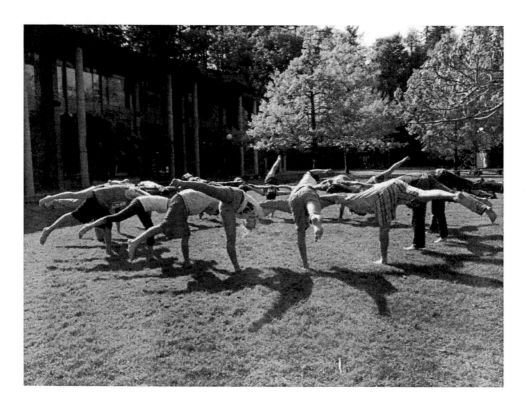

56. diamond dogs (7)

DESCR: Participants start on all fours, in one or more long lines, facing one another backwards, ready to come up into downward-facing dog.
CAUTIONS:
CALLING: "Exhale, curl the toes and come into down dog. Inhale, lift your right foot, finding partner's right foot (this should be a diagonal line across and between your two bodies). Pressing your legs against one another, raising the feet up to the top together, making a nice diamond shape with your legs. Exhale, bring your foot back down. Repeat on other side... Inhale, bend both knees, coming to the ground. Exhale, sink into child's pose."
NOTES:
SLANG NAMES: "Wonder dogs," "dynamo dogs."
RELATED POSES: See also, pose #107, diamond dogs with partial (1-person) levitation.

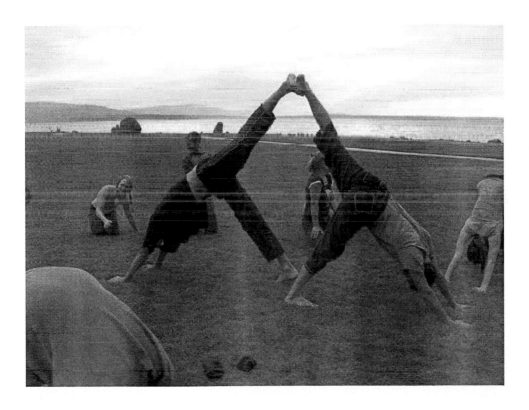

57. side dogs (7)

DESCR: Participants start on all fours, in a line, all facing the same direction, ready to come up into down dogs.
CAUTIONS:
CALLING: "Exhale, everyone, curl your toes and come up into down dog. Everyone but the person in the middle of the line, inhale, lift your inside leg up into the air. Exhale, bring that leg down toward the center, resting on the hip, sacrum, or glute of your neighbor on the side closest to the middle of the group shape. Breathing here. If you like, inhale your inside arm up toward the sky and look down the line at the other dogs. Breathing here. Exhale, bring the hand back down. Inhale, foot back up. Exhale, foot back down to the ground. Inhale, bend both knees, sinking to all fours. Exhale, breathing back to child's pose. Everyone roll one place over down the line, or everyone turn around, and we'll try it again..."
NOTES:
VARIATIONS: Person in the middle can be in child's pose, or on all fours, instead of down-dog, to make this pose easier for the side-dogs, or if the side-dogs are children.
SLANG NAMES: "Fire hydrant dogs," "sidecar dogs," "3-dog," "5-dog," etc. "3-dog day," "3-dog night."

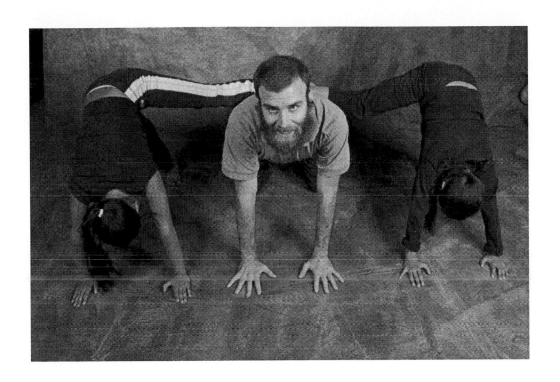

58. dandelion (7)

DESCR: One person in child's pose (referred to as 'the ladybug'). Two people in partner half-moon with bottom hand resting on one shoulder of the person in child's pose. Dancer bigtop (pose #25) with the dancers' top hands to top hands of partner half-moon, gently lifting them.

CAUTIONS: Don't press directly on the spine of the person in the child's pose. Stay on the shoulders and either side of the spine.

CALLING: "Alright, who wants to be the ladybug? Okay, come on down into child's pose. Who wants to be in partner half-moon? Okay, the two of you, with one hand of the child's pose around your inside ankle, slowly lean forward and place your hand on one shoulder of the person in child's pose. Other hand to the sky, overlapping your top hand with your partner's top hand. Now everybody else, gather around and come into dancer bigtop, pressing the hands up in the middle. Breathing here. Inhale, lifting up off the top. Exhale, arm behind. And now the other side. Partner half-moons switch sides and the dancers switch to the other arm and leg. Excellent. Who wants to be the next ladybug?"

NOTES:

VARIATIONS: Stack as many warrior III's, or partner warrior III's, as you like behind the partner half-moon. This is referred to as 'lengthening the stem.'

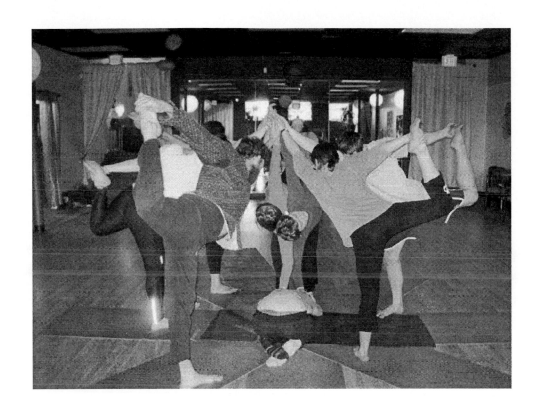

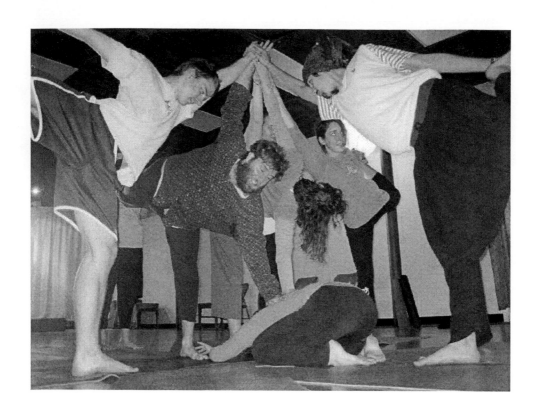

59. spider (7)

DESCR: Partners alternate feet-to-feet and back-to-back, seated in straddle in one or more long lines.
CAUTIONS: Be gentle. Check in with the person on the bottom.
CALLING: "If you're on the inside of the spider, exhale forward to partner's arms or shoulders. If you're on the outside of the spider, inhale your arms up over your head behind you. If you're flexible enough, you may be able to connect inside-to-inside partners and outside-to-outside partners. Breathing here. From there, if you're flexible enough, you can reach through and make a diagonal connection with the hands and arms of the neighbor two people behind you (if you're on the outside of the spider) or two people in front of you (if you're on the inside of the spider). Breathing here. And then slowly coming back up and out."
NOTES:
SLANG NAMES: "Spider arms," "eek! there's a spider on my cruise ship."
RELATED POSES: See also, pose #39, ship at sea.

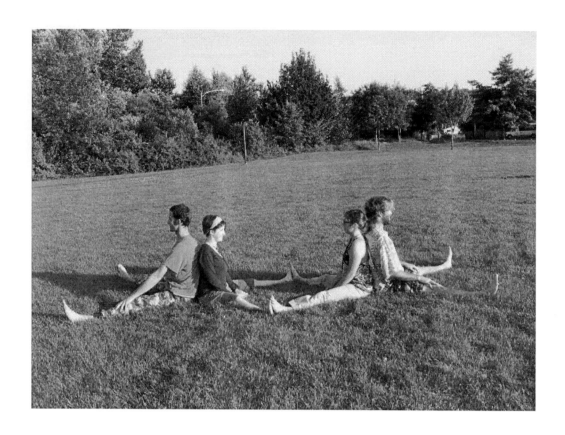

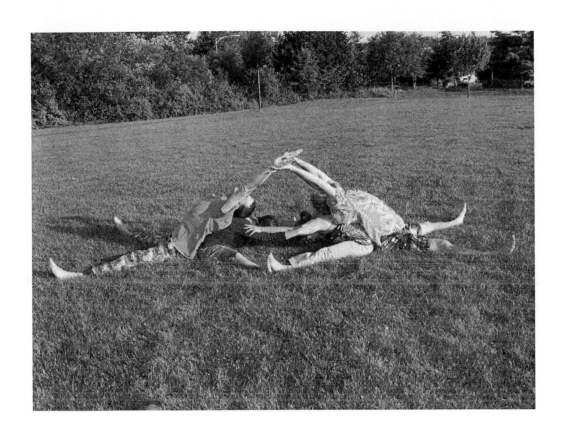

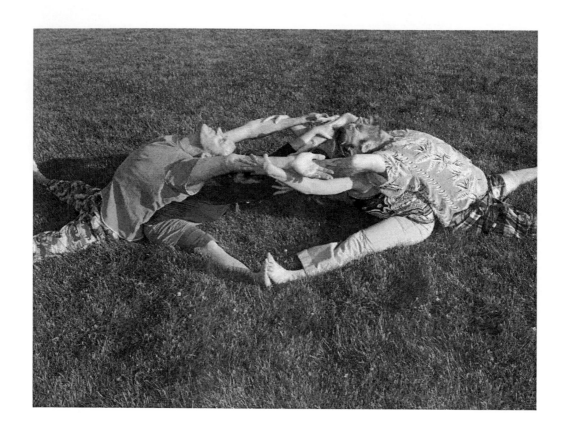

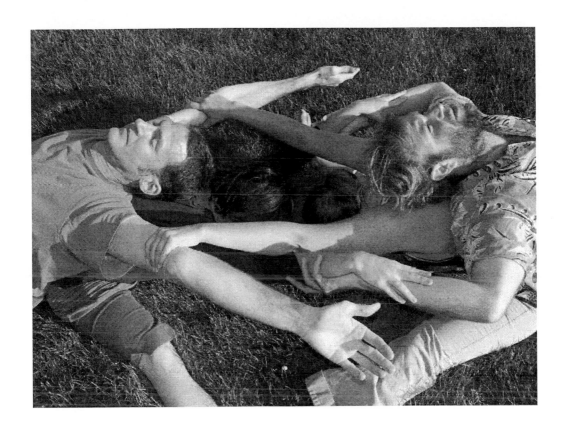

60. short grass, tall grass (7)

DESCR: Trivial pursuit pie with partner-facing straddles. Inner ring, facing out, with backs together in the center, hips to hips, feet spread apart, legs touching or resting next to neighbor's legs. Outer ring, facing the center.
CAUTIONS:
CALLING: "Feet to partner's feet, reach straight across to find partner's right hand or wrist. Inhale, lengthen the spine. Exhale, left hand over the top toward the right, grabbing ahold of diagonal neighbor's hand if it's safe and comfortable. Breathing here. Inhale, back up, switching hands. Exhale, right hand over the top toward the left, grabbing ahold of diagonal neighbor's hand if it's safe and comfortable. Breathing here. Inhale, back up to center. Exhale, rest."
NOTES: Inner ring facing out gets a different stretch than outer ring facing in.
VARIATIONS: Twinkle all the hands up toward the sky. Third layer can provide assist on second layer (outer ring) by gently placing one hand on the hip, second hand on the shoulder, and applying light pressure.
SLANG NAMES: "Grass-in-the-wind for 12," "grass-in-the-wind carousel," "short grass and tall grass blowin' in the wind together," "trivial pursuit pie with partner-facing straddles."
RELATED POSES: See also, pose #20, trivial pursuit pie carousel spin, pose #43, grass-in-the-wind, and pose #86, grass-in-the-wind hexagon.

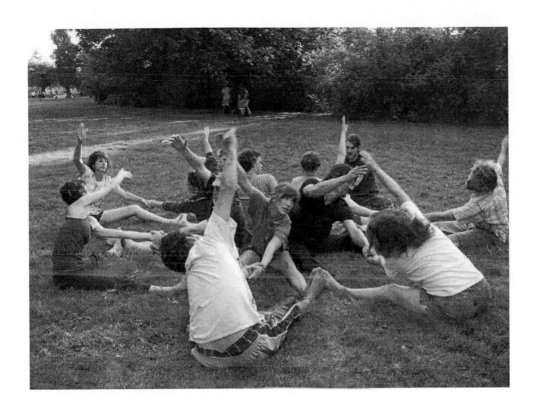

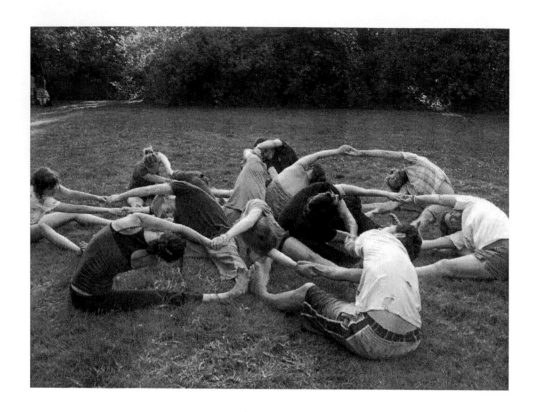

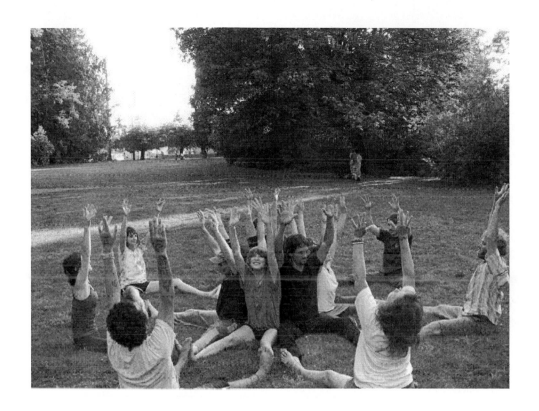

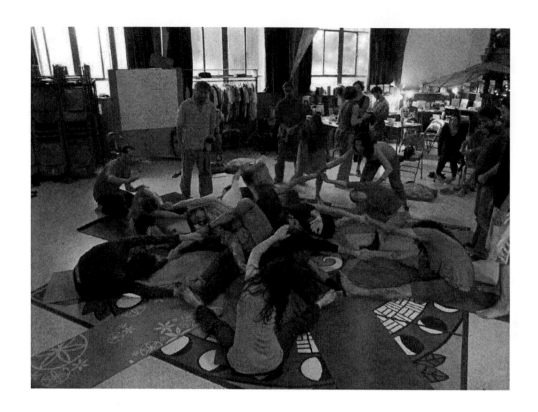

61-67. CLASSIC SEQUENCE #4: partner warrior fractal (7)

61. partner warrior I (7)
62. partner warrior II (7)
63. partner reverse warrior (7)
64. partner straddle hang (7)
65. partner ankle grab (7)
65. partner same side twist (8)
66. partner opposite side twist (8)
67. partner triangle pose (7)

DESCR: Participants stand in a circle, in pairs, looking towards the center of the group shape. Partner warrior I, partner warrior II, partner reverse, partner warrior II, partner straddle hang, partner ankle grab, partner same side twist, partner opposite side twist, partner warrior II, partner triangle, partner warrior II, pull to center, small circle, step back with opposite foot. Repeat sequence on other side with new partner (the next neighbor around the circle).
CAUTIONS:
CALLING: "Inside foot forward. Inside arm around partner's waist, outside arm to the sky, bend that front knee for partner warrior I. Bring your palm to neighbor's palm to connect with the group. Then switch your arms for partner warrior II, overlapping your hands with your partner in front and in back. Optional reach straight or diagonal across to connect with another pair. Flip the front hand over and inhale back to reverse warrior. Optional reach across to connect with another pair. Exhale forward to warrior II. Rotate the feet so they're facing straight away from your partner, who is now behind you. Exhale, folding forward down to your own ankles. Inhale, lift and straighten the spine for monkeyback pose. Exhale, forward, looking between your legs to find partner behind you. Find partner's hands, wrists, forearms, or shoulders. Breathing here. See if you can reach through to find partner's ankles, calves, or shins. Inhale, lift and straighten the spine for monkeyback pose. Exhale, off to the side, for partner same side twist. Same side twist again on the other side. Optional reach across at a diagonal to another pair. Exhale, off to the side, for partner opposide side twist. Opposite side twist again on the other side. Optional reach across at a diagonal to another pair. Back to center. Rest. Then rotate the feet back toward the original center, coming into partner warrior II. Straighten the front leg and sweep down into partner triangle, reaching across to find partner's ankle or shin. Option of taking the top arm (together with

your partner's top arm) forward toward the center to connect with the rest of the group. Inhale up. Warrior II. Reach your hand into the center. Find a matching hand. Pull to the center. And step back into warrior I with a new partner on the other side..."

NOTES:

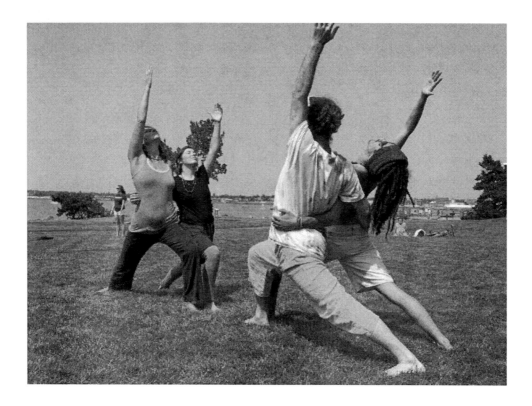

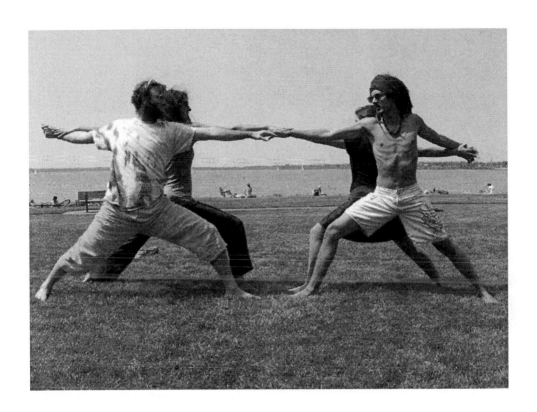

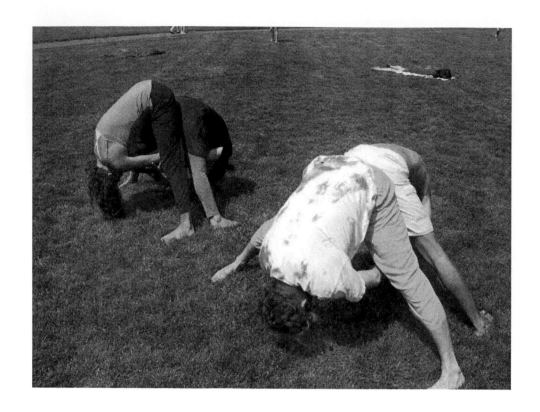

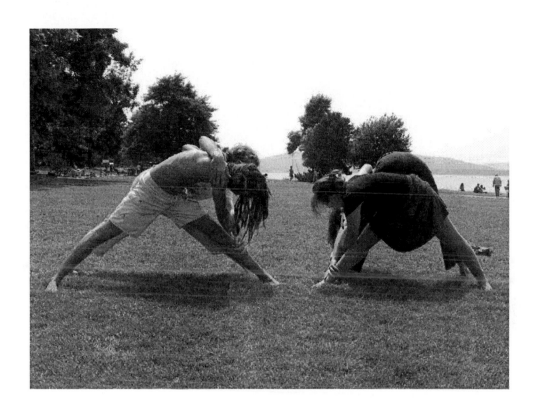

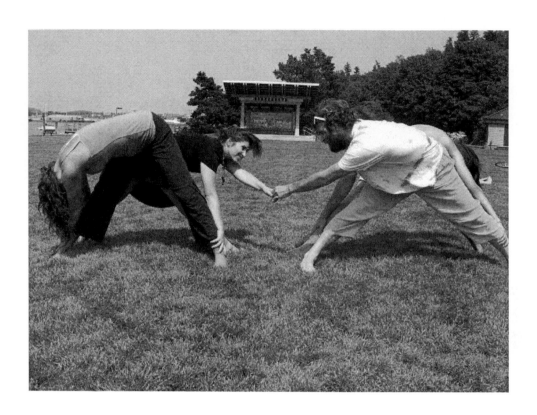

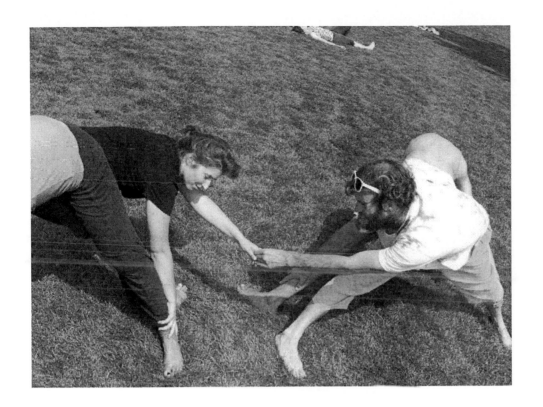

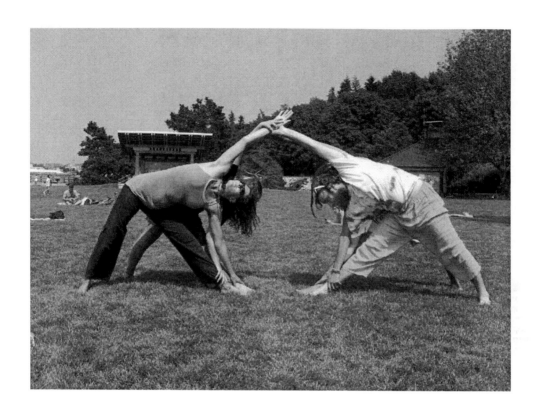

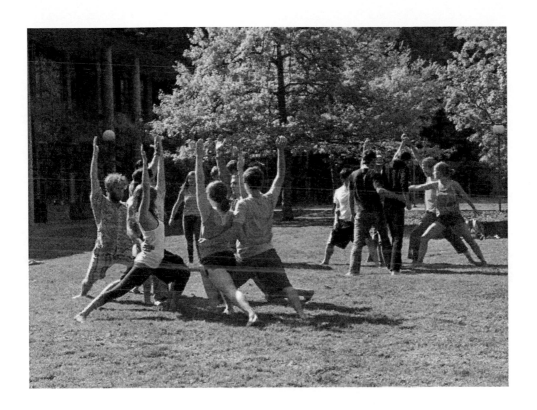

68. side-reclining buddha wheel (7)

DESCR: Participants lay in a circle, with heads toward the center.

CAUTIONS: Don't pull too hard. Check in with your neighbor. Go slowly. Don't lift the foot high up into the air in a way that might be awkward for your neighbor's knee. Just slowly, gently pull back in a way that keeps the leg horizontal. Three people is possible, but not generally recommended, only for those who are extremely flexible.

CALLING: "Now roll over onto your right side and reach your right arm into the middle. Now curl your fingertips together with the rest of your group. Now bend your left knee and with your left hand grad ahold of your own left ankle or shin and give yourself a little warm-up quad stretch. Now reach forward for your neighbor's left foot in front of you. Grab ahold and gently start to pull back, checking in with that person to see how they are doing. Breathing here. Slowly letting go. Rolling back to center, and we'll try the other side..."

NOTES: You may feel the stretch and an opening in the shoulder and arm braced against the ground as much as you do in the leg. The fewer the people, the farther the reach and the more intense the stretch.

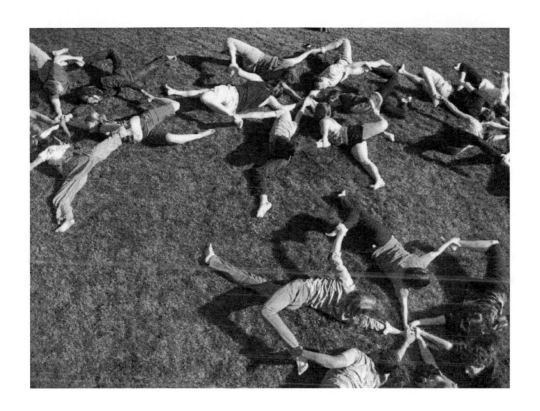

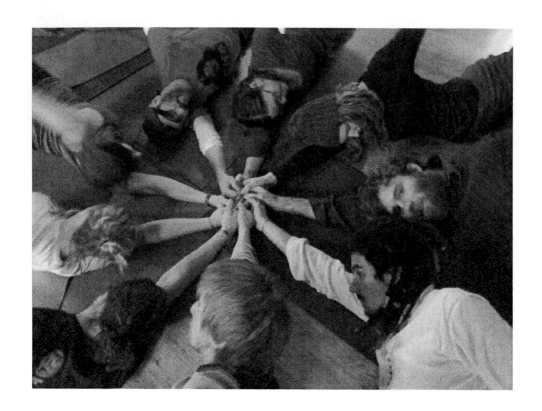

69. baddha konasana clover thai massage twist assist (7)

DESCR: Participants sit in small groups, soles of the feet together, knees folded out to the sides. Assistants stand directly behind them.
CAUTIONS: Be gentle.
CALLING: "Inhale, lengthen the spine. Exhale, folding forward to neighbors' feet. Then, leaving your left hand in place on neighbor's foot to your left, inhale, lengthen and straighten your spine. Exhale, take your right hand behind you. If you're behind them offering support, gently take one hand to the hand and one hand behind the shoulder. Gently coming back to center, and we'll try the other side."
NOTES:
VARIATIONS: Those assisting from behind may find it easier or more comfortable from a half-kneeling position. The knee of the person giving the assist may also be used on the back of the shoulder.

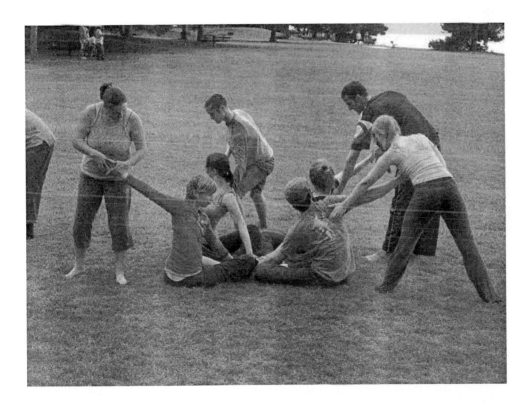

70. baddha konasana clover thai massage backwalk (7)

DESCR: Half the participants per group sit in a circle, soles of the feet together, knees folded out to the sides. The other half per group sits directly behind the first group, with knees bent, feet on the backs of the first group. Holding wrists from behind, gently walk the feet up and down the back.
CAUTIONS:
CALLING: "Inner circle, bring your hands behind you. Outer circle, with knees bent, reach forward and find the wrists of the person in front of you. Slowly, gently walk your feet up and down the back, staying on either side of the spine."
NOTES: For the person receiving massage, keep the spine straight. For the person giving massage, don't pull the person backwards or off-center. Bend the knees and scoot forward if necessary.

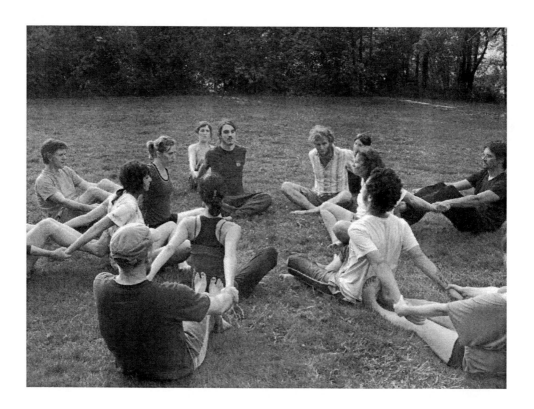

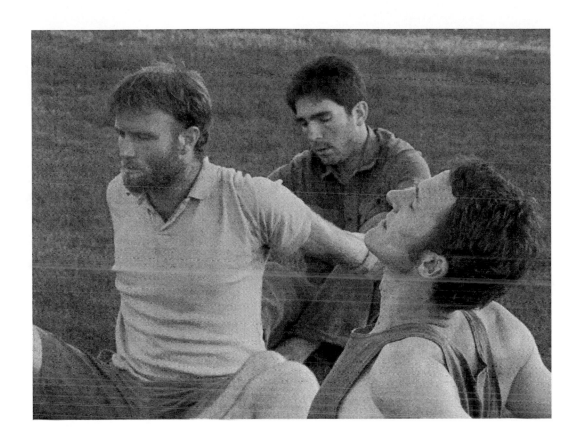

71. dog-back (7)

DESCR: One person comes into down dog. Second person stands, with feet outside of first person's hands, facing away, then gently sits back, then lays back all the way on the first person's back. Third person can gently pull on the hands or the wrists of the second person from behind the pair.

CAUTIONS: Do not lift someone who is more than 25 pounds heavier than you are. Do not sit so high on the down-dog that you fall off the back when you lean back.

CALLING: "So, one person coming into down dog. Second person starts with their feet on either side of the hands of the person in down dog, facing away. And then gently sit back against the back of the person in down dog. And then lay all the way back, and let your arms go up over the top. Breathing here. A third person can come around behind and gently lengthen out the second. Breathing here. And then slowly come back up."

NOTES: Third person is optional. Second person can adjust their height relative to the first person. If you sit lower, it's sturdier and less intense. If you sit higher, more of you can drape off the back end, giving a more intense back bend and chest opening.

VARIATIONS: If second person is extremely flexible, they can reach back and grab calves, ankles, or shins of the first person. Second person can gently lift their feet off the ground. Second person can overlap their feet together with legs wrapped around the torso of the first person. Third person assist can also crouch or squat. Third person assist can also gently press down on Achilles or heels of person in down-dog.

SLANG NAMES: "Dog-back riding," "dog-o-matic back stretcher."

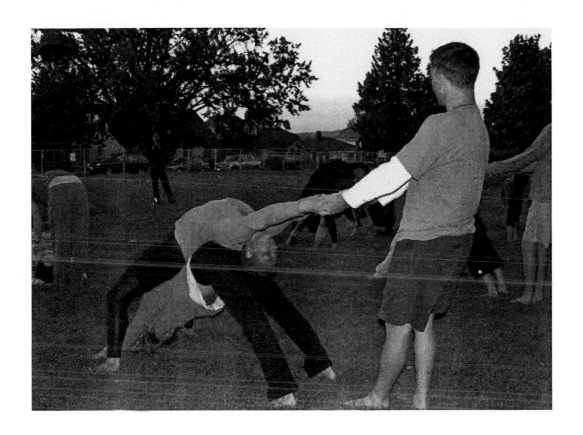

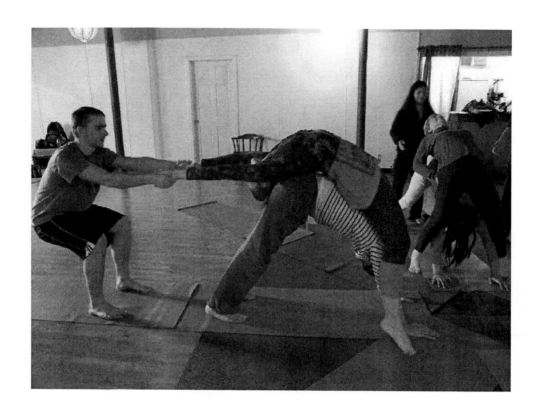

72. 4-hand massage for child's pose (7)

DESCR: One person in child's pose. Two others on either side (one in front, one in back).
CAUTIONS: Don't press directly on the spine of the person in the child's pose. Stay on the shoulders and on either side of the back.
CALLING: "Starting on all fours, sinking back into child's pose, and then one person on either side, gently massaging and pressing out the back."
NOTES:
VARIATIONS: People giving the massage can reach across to opposite sides, one partner around the second partner's arms. Cross press opposites: one person on hip/ sacrum and opposite shoulder, second person on other hip/ sacrum and opposite shoulder. Shared (double) press: One person's hands on top of the second person's hands. Shared (double) cross press: One person's hands on top of the second person's hands, double press on hip/ sacrum and opposite shoulder, then switch, double press on other hip/ sacrum and opposite shoulder.
SLANG NAMES: "Well-loved inner child," "can we do this all hour?"

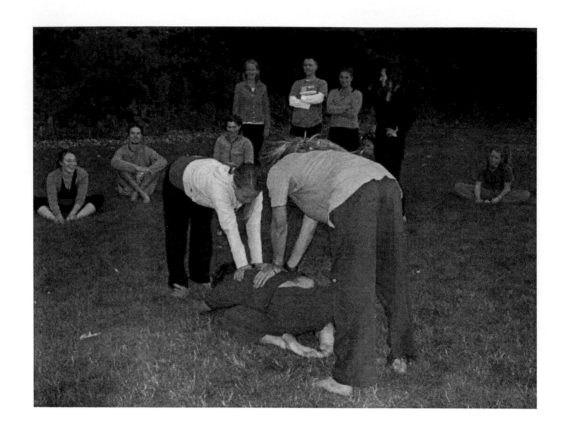

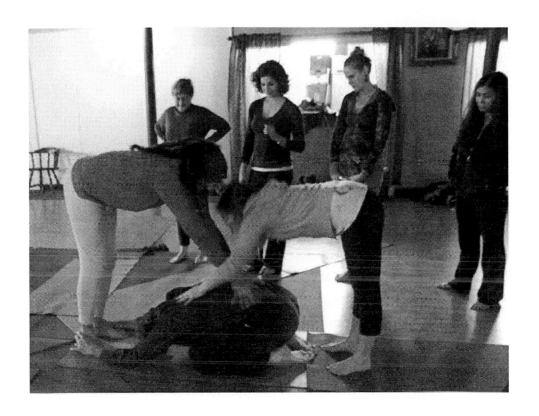

73. dog-back skydive (7)

DESCR: Multiple pairs of dog-back, with heels of downward dogs facing toward the center.
CAUTIONS: Do not lift someone who is more than 25 pounds heavier than you are.
CALLING: "So, starting with all the dogs facing heels to center. Those who are going to be backbending, you can have your feet on either side of the hands of someone in down dog. Then gently sit back, and lay back. Once you lay all the way back and are feeling comfortable, you can take your hands to neighbor's hands, wrists, forearms, biceps or shoulders. Breathing here. Inhale, slowly come back up. Exhale, counterpose with a forward fold, or rest in child's pose."
NOTES:

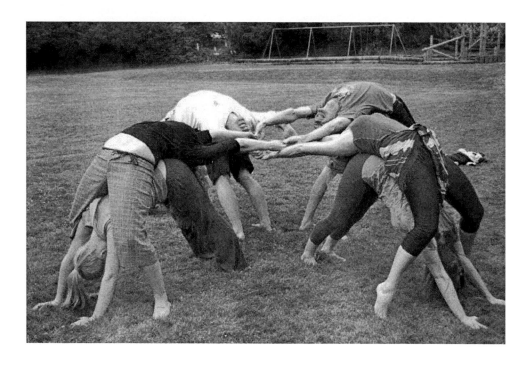

74. crab cross lift (7)

DESCR: Participants sit in a small circle of 3 or 4, as in baddha konasana clover, soles of the feet together, knees folded out to the sides.
CAUTIONS:
CALLING: "Lift your right leg, and take it further to the right, resting your foot across neighbor's hip, scooting in to make sure your heel is well past the edge of your neighbor's leg. Now lift your left leg, and do the same thing, place it further to the left, resting on neighbor's hip. Turn your hands around backwards so fingertips are facing away from the center of the shape. One, two, three, lift."
NOTES:
VARIATIONS: Once lifted, swing the shape around in circles. Switch directions. Crab-walk the whole larger shape around. Lift pelvises one at a time around the shape in a wave.
SLANG NAMES: "Leg cabin," "leg cabin lift."

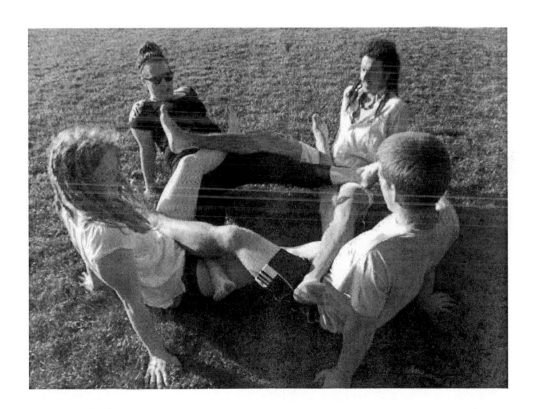

75. crab cross tetrahedron lift (8)

DESCR: Participants sit in a small circle of 3 or 4, as in baddha konasana clover, soles of the feet together, knees folded out to the sides.
CAUTIONS:
CALLING: "Lift your right leg, and take it further to the right, resting your foot across neighbor's hip, scooting in to make sure your heel is well past the edge of your neighbor's leg. Now lift your left leg, and do the same thing, place it further to the left, resting on neighbor's hip. Turn your hands around backwards so fingertips are facing away from the center of the shape. One, two, three, lift. Now take the top (right) foot, up toward the sky, straightening the right leg, pressing into neighbors' right feet when you get to the top. Breathing here. Slowly lower back down. Switch sides and repeat."
NOTES:
VARIATIONS: Once lifted, swing the shape around in circles. Switch directions. Crab-walk the whole larger shape around. Lift pelvises one at a time around the shape in a wave.
SLANG NAMES: "Lifted pyramid," "floating pyramid," "levitating pyramid," "crabby pyramid."

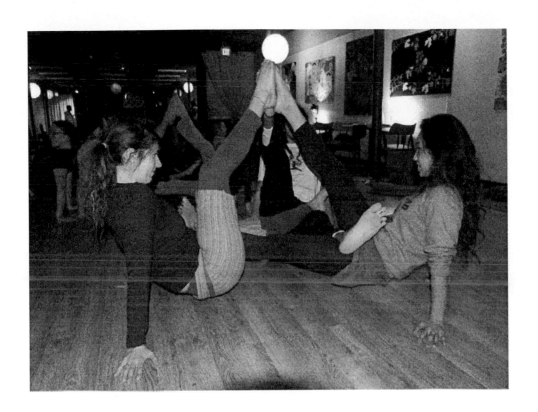

76. acro-on-the boat deck (7)

DESCR: For example: 3-person boat, 3 bases, 3 flyers, (with optional 3 spotters).
CAUTIONS: Do not lift someone who is more than 25 pounds heavier than you are. Practice acro-yoga in pairs first with plenty of space around before attempting to combine pairs into acro-on-the boat deck. Careful not to bonk heads.
CALLING: "Let's have the boat pose come up first. Okay, excellent. Next, the bases can crawl underneath with their heads toward the middle, with one head of space in between them, and then raise their hands up through the holes in between the arms and legs of the boat pose. Next, flyers can find yourself a base, and come on up."
NOTES:
VARIATIONS: Flyers take one hand to center, other hand to center, both hands to center, one hand to neighbor's shoulder. Flyers take hands to head or crown chakra of people in boat pose, flyers place hands on feet of boat poses. This is known as 'all hands on deck.' If flyers have their hands up on the feet of the boat pose, bases can also take their hands to the wrists of the boat pose and 'row the boat.'

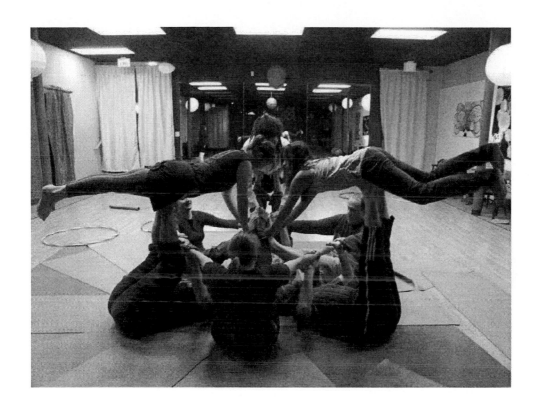

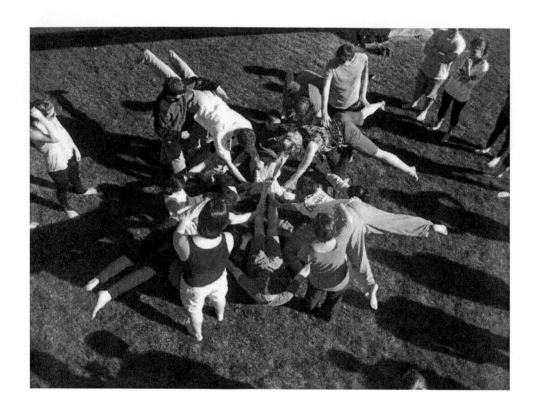

77. shaolin horse hamstrings (7)

DESCR: One person in horse stance, two others on either side with one heel resting in the nook of the elbow of the person in horse stance.
CAUTIONS:
CALLING: "Inhale, lengthen the spine. Exhale, fold your outside arm over the top, and reach toward your foot, keeping the top shoulder rolled back. Breathing here. Inhale, arm up off the top. Exhale, arm behind. Bending the knee, bringing the foot back down, and rotate."
NOTES:
VARIATIONS: If you're feeling flexible, you can give the person in horse stance a playful little tug on the ear.
SLANG NAMES: "Shaolin horse stance leg stretch ear pull."

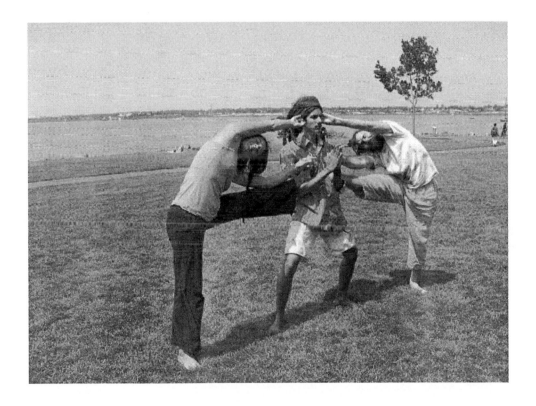

78. zipper legs arm-wrestler leanaway (7)

DESCR: Participants sit in two long lines, facing one another, with every other person facing in alternating directions, like a zipper. Feet next to neighbor's hips.
CAUTIONS:
CALLING: "So we're gonna sit in one long line, facing one another, with every other person facing in alternating directions, like a zipper. Starting with your legs next to your neighbors' legs on either side, feet next to neighbors' hips on either side. Now, bend your right knee and wrap your right leg around the right leg of the person in front of you, facing you, sitting just to your right. Now, bend your left knee and wrap your left leg around the left leg of the person in front of you, facing you, sitting just to your left. Now, scoot forward so you're nice and snug, and your feet are well past neighbors' hips. Now, stick your hands out in front of you, and grab ahold of the hands of the people sitting across from you with an arm-wrestle grip. Inhale, everyone lengthen. Exhale, lean back. Breathing here. Inhale, back up to center."
NOTES:
VARIATIONS: Holding hands, swing around as a group in figure 8's. Arm-wrestle. Smile. Laugh.
SLANG NAMES: "Arm wrestler's dream," "arm wrestler's nightmare," "tantric arm-wrestling convention," "leglock line arm wrestler leanaway."

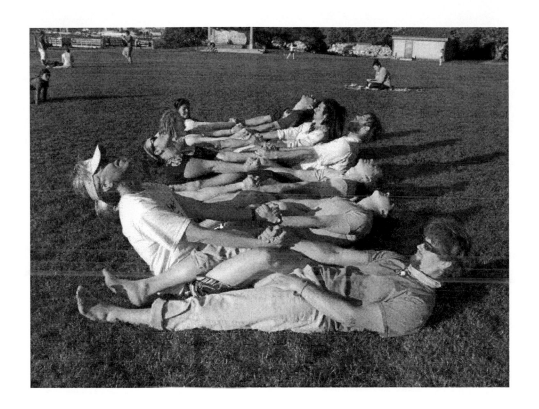

79. zipper legs crab-lift (8)

DESCR: Participants sit in one long line with knees bent, hips open to the sides, legs intertwined with their neighbors.
CAUTIONS:
CALLING: "So we're gonna sit in one long line, facing one another, with every other person facing in alternating directions, like a zipper. Starting with your legs next to your neighbors' legs on either side, feet next to neighbors' hips on either side. Now, bend your right knee and wrap your right leg around the right leg of the person in front of you, facing you, sitting just to your right. Now, bend your left knee and wrap your left leg around the left leg of the person in front of you, facing you, sitting just to your left. Now scoot forward so you're nice and snug, and your feet are well past neighbors' hips. Turning your hands backwards, place them on the ground behind you. On the count of three, we're all going to lift ourselves up. Ready? 1, 2, 3... Lift. Breathing here. And then slowly coming back down. Rest."
NOTES:
VARIATIONS: Swing the lifted shape around in figure 8's. Lift the pelvises one at a time down the line, making a wave.
SLANG NAMES: "Leglock line crab lift."

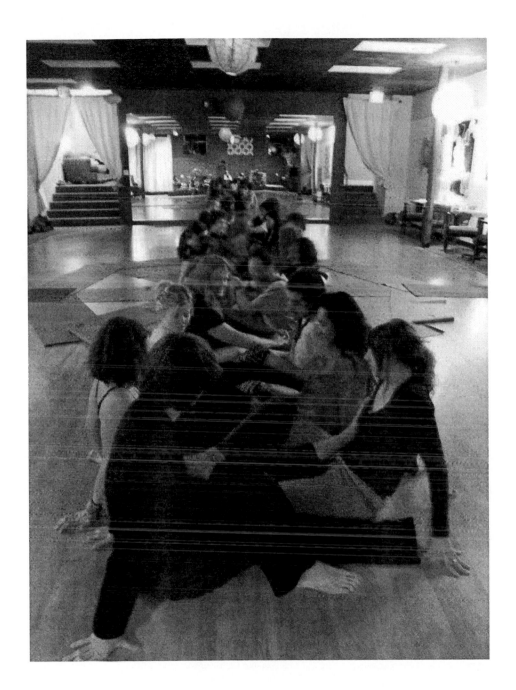

80. pigeon pairs (7)

DESCR: Participants come into pigeon pose with a partner.
CAUTIONS:
CALLING: "Finding a partner, you can come into pigeon pose, nesting the foot of your bent (forward) leg together with your partner's foot. Inside arm around partner's shoulder. You can then raise your outside arm, bringing your palm to neighbor's palm or your hand to neighbor's shoulder. Breathing here. Slowly coming back out and switching sides."
NOTES: You can press into the palms to help lengthen the spine. You can switch legs and sides with your immediate partner, or, by moving around the circle to a new partner, the next neighbor around the circle on the other side.
SLANG NAMES: "Happy pigeon family," "partner pigeon fractal."
RELATED POSES: See also, pose #53, pigeon circle, and pose #54, pigeon huddle.

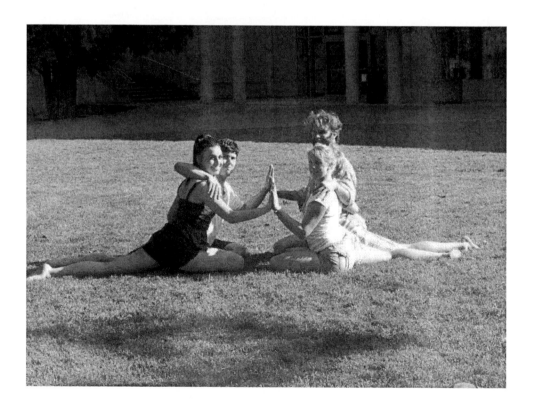

81. air traffic control (7)

DESCR: Multiple pairs of acro bases and flyers cross hands with neighbors.
CAUTIONS: Do not lift someone who is more than 25 pounds heavier than you are. Practice acro-yoga in pairs first with plenty of space around before attempting to combine pairs into air traffic control. Careful not to bonk heads.
CALLING: "So, who's feeling strong and sturdy? Let's have a few brave volunteers lying on their backs with their heads near one another, with one head's distance apart from one another. And then, who's feeling light and airy? People who want to fly can align themselves with a base. Bases bend your knees, feet to flyers' hip bones. Palms to palms, and leg press them on up. Steady your balance here. Breathing. Flyers, once you're feeling steady, you can try taking your hands to the hands of the neighboring base, one hand at a time. And the other hand. Nice. Breathing here. And slowly coming back to your original base. And gently back down. Flyers, you can shake your base's legs and give them a little massage and press on the feet."
NOTES.
VARIATIONS: Flyers raise one hand to the middle. Flyers raise one hand to neighbor's shoulder.

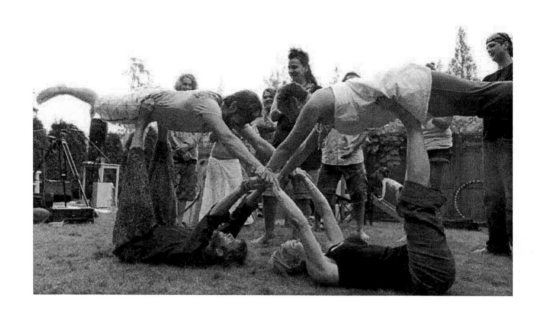

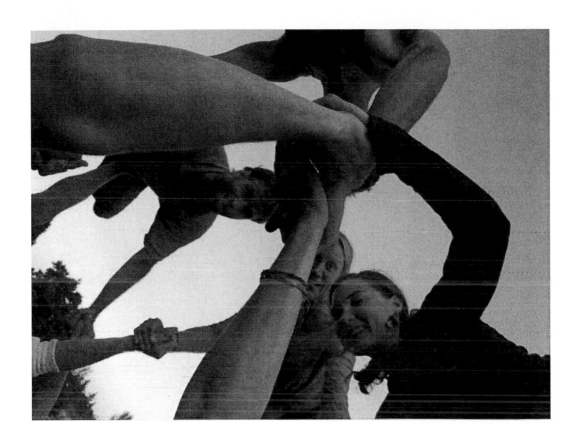

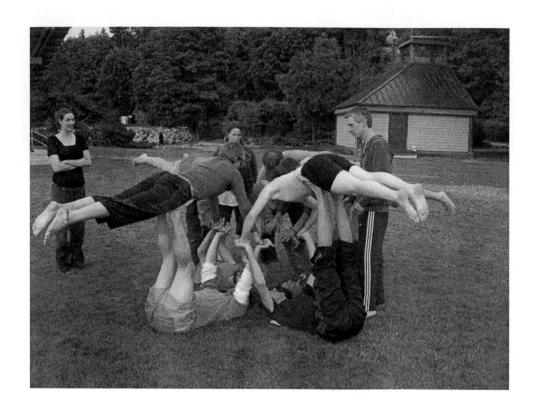

82. jellyfish hip and sacrum massage collective (7)

DESCR: Participants lay in a circle, with feet to the center. Start holding neighbor's hands.
CAUTIONS:
CALLING: "Inhale, raise your right foot and leg high up into the sky. Exhale, roll that leg across your body to the left, placing your foot against the back of neighbor's sacrum. Gently press around on neighbor's hip, sacrum, and glute. Inhale, right leg back to the sky. Exhale, leg down to center and rest. And we'll try it again on the other side. Inhale, raise your left foot and leg high up into the sky..."
NOTES:

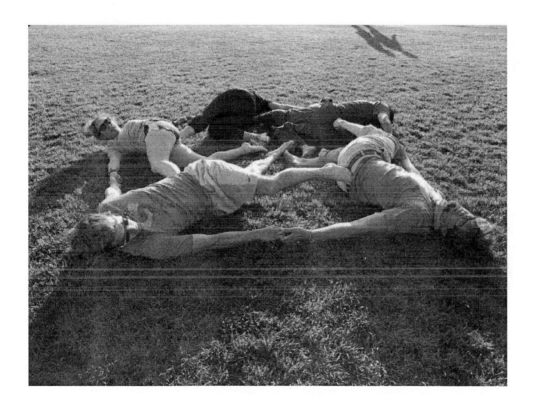

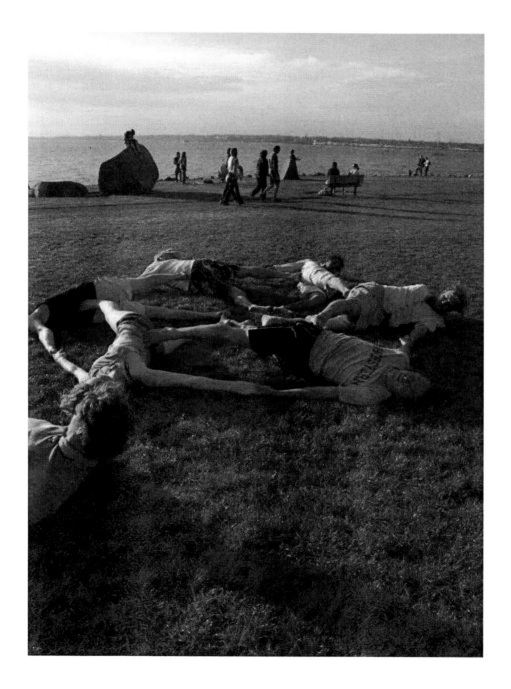

83. lunge circle (7)

DESCR: Participants stand in a circle, facing the center, slightly wider than shoulder to shoulder apart.
CAUTIONS: Keep front knee over ankle.
CALLING: "Starting with palms to neighbor's palms, step your right foot back into a lunge, raising your right heel off the ground. Bending the front knee and sinking down into the lunge as far as is comfortable and safe. Breathing here. Stepping forward and we'll try the other side."
NOTES:
VARIATIONS: Gently send energy around the circle through the hands. Make waves with the arms. Push back and forth on neighbors.
RELATED POSES: This pose sequences well with pyramid circle. Do lunge circle and pyramid circle on right side. Bend front knee, step forward. Do lunge circle and pyramid circle on left side. Bend front knee, step forward.

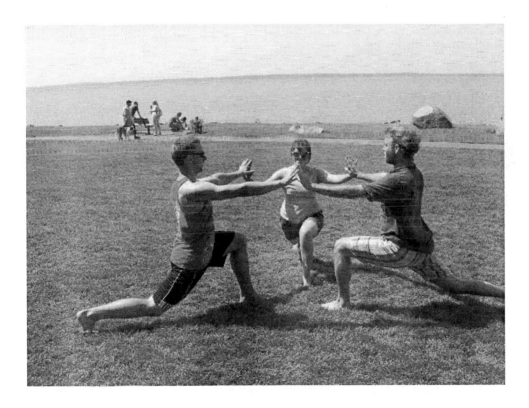

84. pyramid circle (8)

DESCR: Participants start in a circle, facing the center. Standing slightly wider than shoulder-to-shoulder apart, palms to neighbors' palms.
CAUTIONS:
CALLING: "Starting palms to neighbors' palms, we're all going to step our right foot back into warrior stance. Now exhale, gently reaching forward towards neighbors' shoulders to come into pyramid pose, bringing your forehead toward your shin. Breathing here. Inhale, slowly come back up. Bend the front knee, stepping forward, and we'll try it again on the other side."
NOTES:
RELATED POSES: This pose sequences well with lunge circle. Do lunge circle and pyramid circle on right side. Bend front knee, step forward. Do lunge circle and pyramid circle on left side. Bend front knee, step forward.

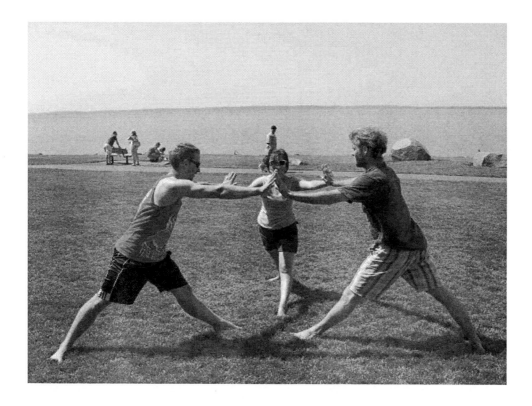

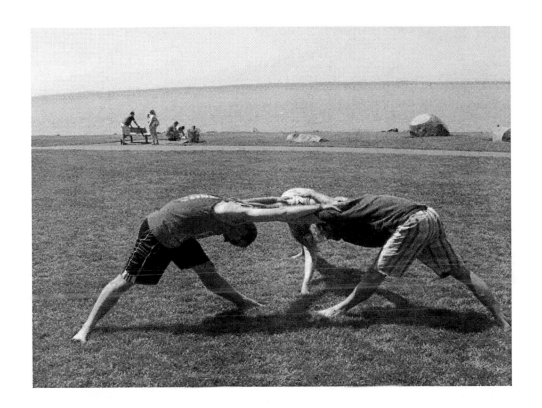

85. reclining hero family takes the train (7)

DESCR: Participants start kneeling in one long line ('the train'). One at a time, people lay back into reclining hero pose on top of the person behind them.
CAUTIONS:
CALLING: "Kneeling in a line, starting with your right hand up in the air. Choo, choo! Now, one at a time, lower back to rest your head on the stomach of the person behind you. Breathing here for a while. Inhale, coming back up. Exhale, rest."
NOTES:
VARIATIONS: The person in the very front of the train is the 'conductor.' Any extras behind the conductor who are just kneeling upright and not laying back are 'passengers.' The people laying back flat on one another are 'freight cars.' The person at the end of the line (with their back to the ground and not another person, holding more weight) is the 'baggage car.' And if you add one more child's pose to the very end, that's the 'caboose.' Play with different combinations.

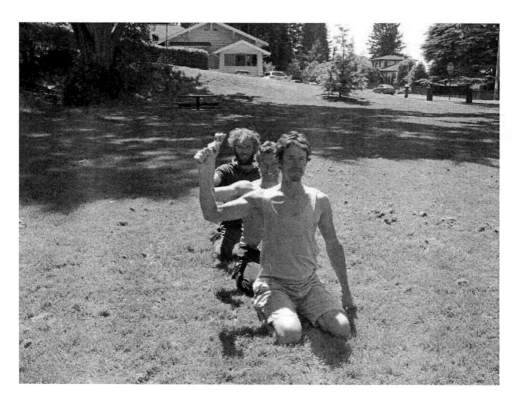

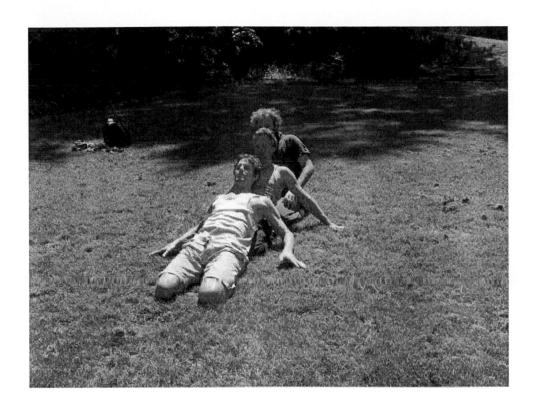

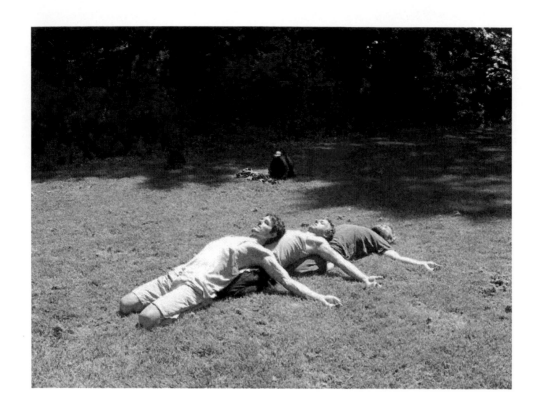

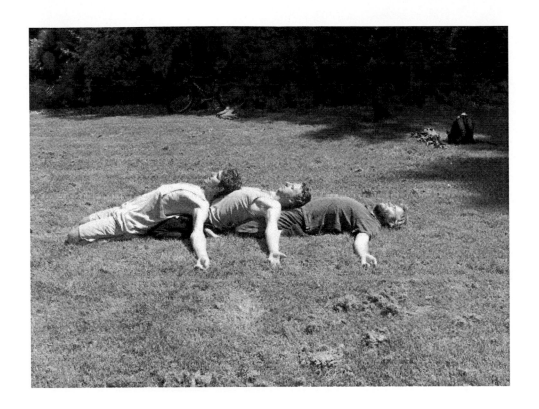

86. grass-in-the-wind hexagon (7)

DESCR: Participants start in 3 partner-facing straddles per hexagon, with one foot to the middle of the hexagon, and one foot to the outside.
CAUTIONS: Don't strain your hamstrings just to reach neighbor's hands. Bend your knees if necessary.
CALLING: "Reach straight across to the partner directly in front of you and grab their right hand or wrist. Inhale, lengthen the spine. Exhale, left hand over the top to the right. 3 of you will have your hands together in the middle. 3 of you will have your hands to the outside. Inhale, back up, and we'll try it again on the other side."
NOTES:
VARIATIONS: Windshield wiper the hands back and forth between the feet in the middle and the feet on the outside. Switch partners and repeat.
RELATED POSES: See also, pose #43, grass-in-the-wind.

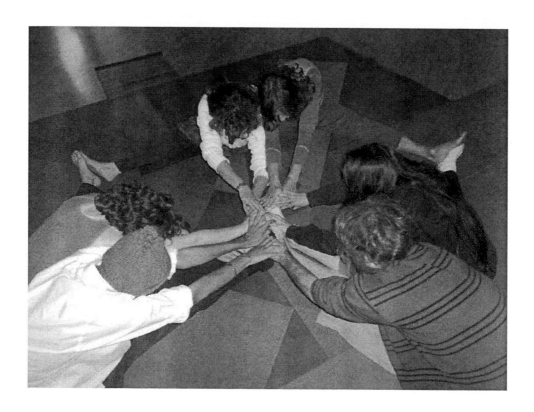

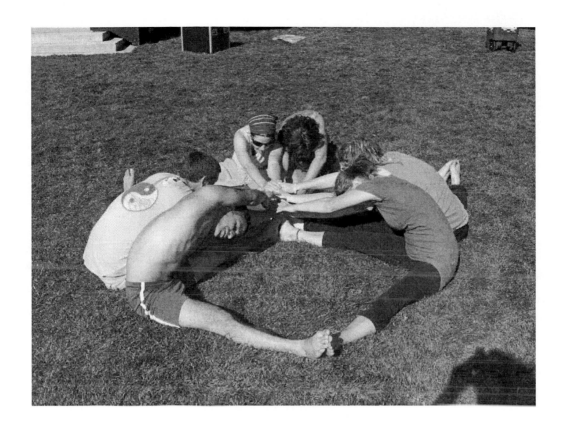

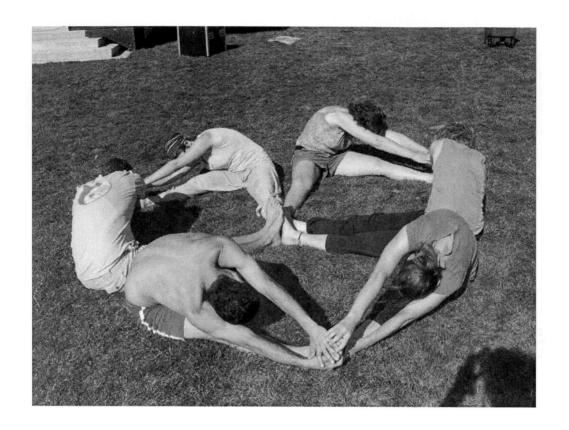

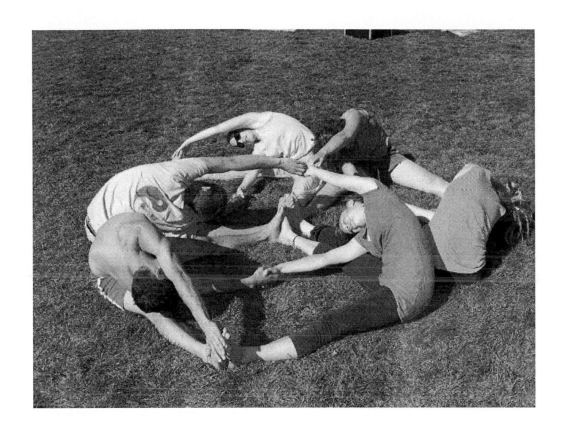

87. trillium reclining heroes and heroines (8)

DESCR: Participants start kneeling in a circle, backs toward the center, with lots of space in between them. Lowering slowly backwards, first onto forearms and elbows, to check the flexibility of the quads and the spacing. Adjusting if necessary, and then all the way back to rest with crowns lightly touching in the center. Take hands to the sides to find neighbor's hands.
CAUTIONS:
CALLING: "Breathing together on the ground. And then, inhale, bringing hands up to the sky and together in the middle. Exhale, lower hands back down to the sides. Repeat. Resting here. And then slowly coming back up and out."
NOTES:
VARIATIONS: quadrillium, pentillium, etc.

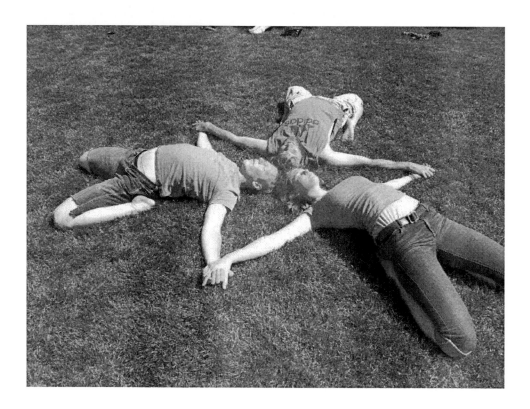

88. yin/ yang straddle plow, seated straddle (8)

DESCR: One person sits in a straddle, with legs in an equilateral triangle. Second person starts with head in between first person's legs and hands on first person's feet or ankles.
CAUTIONS:
CALLING: "Start with one partner seated in a straddle. Second partner can lay on their back with their head in between the feet of the first partner, hands resting on the first partner's ankles. Then, grabbing ahold of the ankles, roll back into plow pose, resting your feet on the backs of your partner's shoulders."
NOTES:
VARIATIONS: Person in plow can start with toes tucked on backs of shoulders, feet on either side of the neck of the person in seated straddle. Breathing here. Second person (in seated straddle) can widen out the legs of the plow into straddle plow, then gently press down on the first person's heels, bringing their feet to the ground. Gently lengthen out the Achilles by pulling on the heels. Bring the feet back up to the shoulders. With both hands on one calf of the person in plow, the plow pose can raise one leg at a time to the sky, in a shoulder-stand variation. Gently lean leg away from seated straddle, opening up the low back. Take the foot low and out to the side. Back up to the shoulder. Switch legs. Repeat. The second person (in seated straddle) can scoot back, giving the plow pose more room. Plow pose can come into Karnipadasana, (knees to ears, bent knees, shins along the floor). Breathing here. Assist can lightly hold on heels. Assist can then come around to the front and sit with their spine gently against the spine of the person who was in Karnipadasana, and is now in plow pose once again. Person seated can stretch their legs out long in front. Hands resting on the hands of the plow pose. Breathing here. Plow pose can come up into shoulder stand, with their spine braced against the person seated with their legs out long. Person in shoulder stand can bend their knees, lowering their feet to dangle over the shoulders of the person who is seated. The person seated can gently grab their ankles. Breathing here. Giving the person in shoulder-stand time to turn their hands over and tuck them under, ready to press up off their neck. Going slowly and communicating clearly. On the count of three, the person who is seated, with their hands around the other person's ankles, can slowly lean forward into a seated forward fold, pulling the person forward and on top of them. Breathing here. The extra weight of the person laying on top of the seated forward fold will help them deepen into it. The person on top can then place their feet on

the ground, and press up into upward-facing wheel. Breathing here. The person who was underneath can carefully crawl out. Voilá! Lowering back down. Rest.

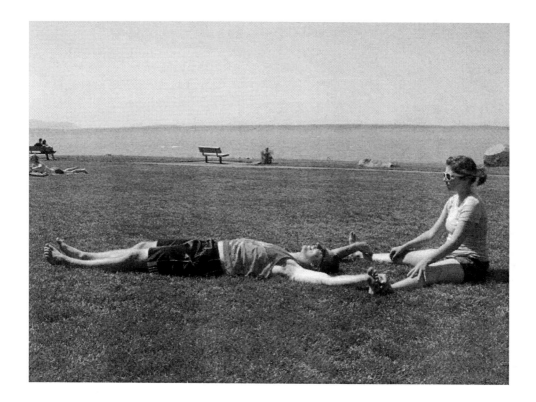

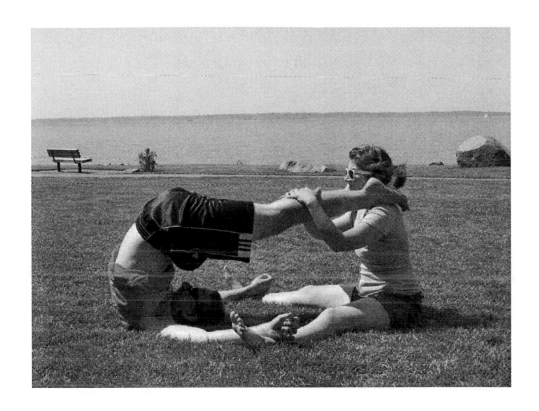

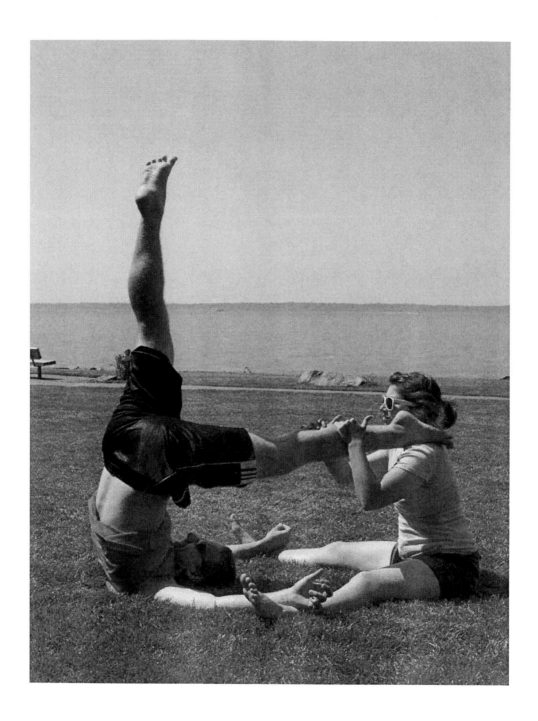

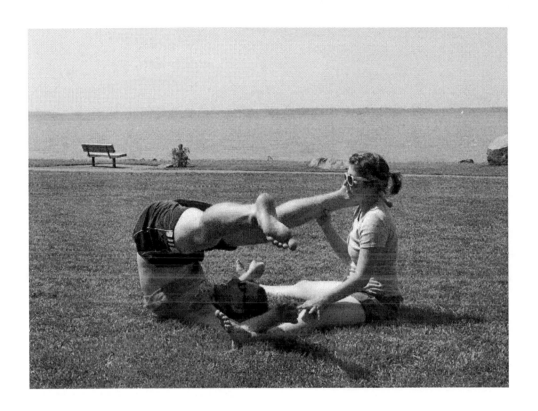

89. grounded swaying palms (8)

DESCR: Start in earth, heart, sky (pose # 10).
CAUTIONS: Don't fall over. Don't push.
CALLING: "Inhale, bring the hands up, over the head. Exhale, hands down toward the ground. When you get to the bottom, see if you can bring your thumbs to the ground. If that's comfortable, see if you can grab neighbors' near ankles on either side. If that's comfortable, see if you can grab neighbors' far ankles. If that's comfortable, see if you can bring your palms to the ground. Without falling in, gently lean in towards the center, bracing yourself against neighbors' arms and shoulders. Now very gently, sway the shape around in a circle. Pause. Now sway the shape around in the other direction. Exhale, rest. And then inhale slowly back up."
NOTES:
SLANG NAMES: "Group palm reading from the earth."

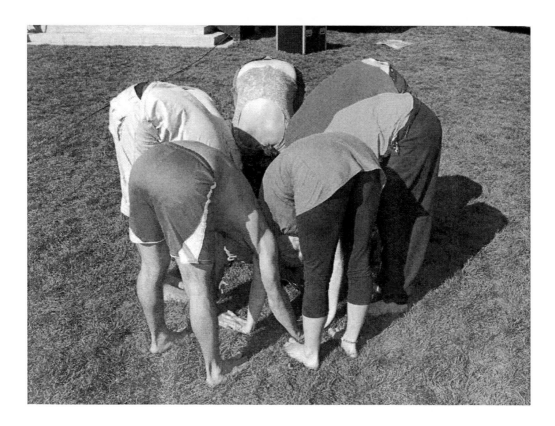

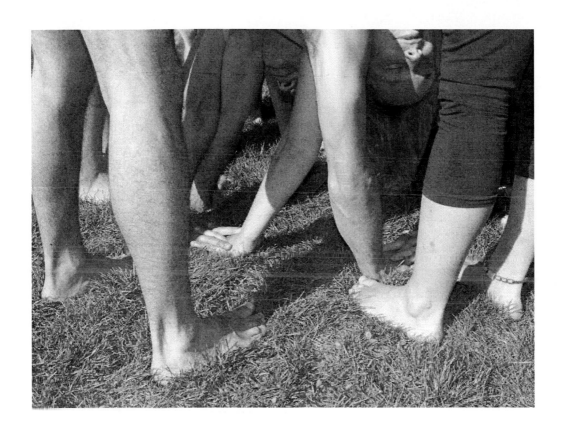

90. standing back-to-back lift (8)

DESCR: Participants stand back-to-back. One person ('the lifter') interlaces their elbows underneath the arms of the second person, widens their stance, and then leans forward to lift the second person up. Breathing here. Coming back down. Switch roles. Repeat.

CAUTIONS: Do not lift someone who is more than 25 pounds heavier than you are. Tell the person being lifted not to jump up on your back. No need to jump, no need to hold yourself up, no need to raise your feet or legs. Just relax and let the person lifting gently bring you off the ground by leaning forward.

CALLING: "Start standing back to back. Interlace your elbows. Decide who is lifting who first. The person doing the lifting, widen your stance. Feet pointing straight ahead, knees wide. Sink down so your hips are below your partner's. Slowly, gently lean forward, lifting your partner off the ground. Breathing here. Once your partner is completely lifted, you can slowly take their hands out to the sides and up over their head. The person being lifted may also rest their head and neck off to one side in between the neck and one shoulder of the lifter. You can lengthen out the liftee's arms. Breathing here. Then slowly coming back down."

NOTES: Usually works best if the person doing the lifting starts out lower than the person being lifted. If you're lifting, keep your knees wide, don't let them sag inward. You can also brace with your forearms against your thighs for more support.

VARIATIONS: Gently shift weight from side to side, adding a little tiny pull on the wrists or forearms if you like. Take both of the liftee's hands, stretch them out the front. Place the liftee's palms together. Liftee takes head to one side, resting in between the neck and shoulder of the lifter. Then the other side. The liftee (if particularly flexible) can bend their knees and tuck their feet into the hip creases of the lifter. If the liftee is particularly acrobatic and monkey-like, the partners can grab hands and the person on top can bend their knees, roll their feet over the top toward the head, and somersault backwards to bring their feet to the ground.

SLANG NAMES: "The green lantern." (Don't ask.)

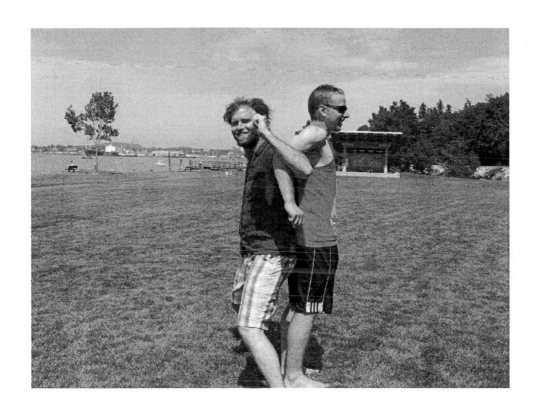

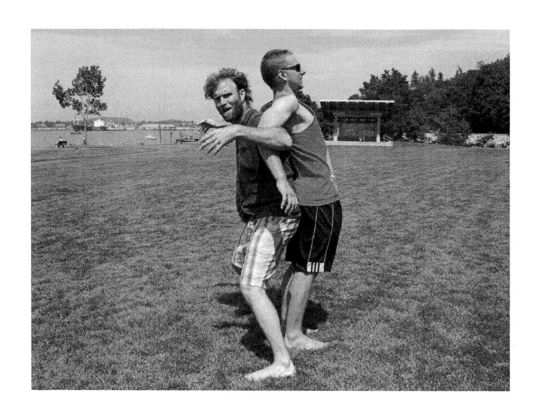

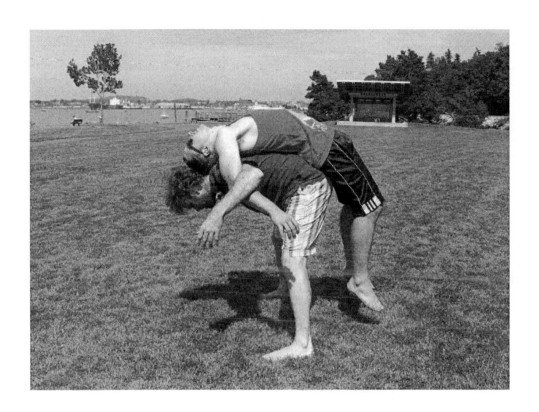

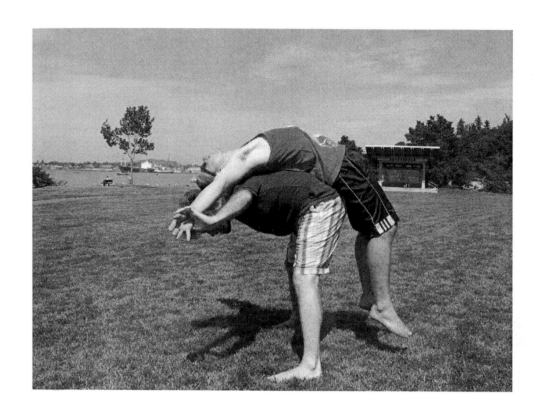

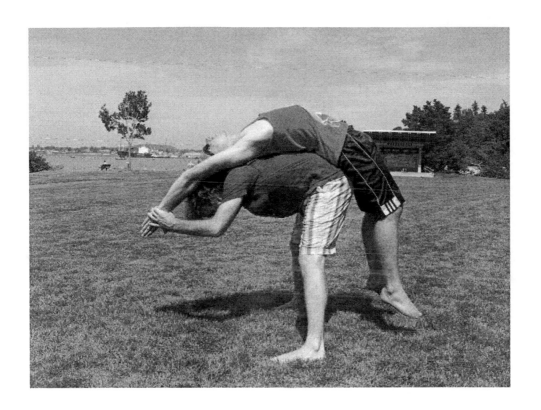

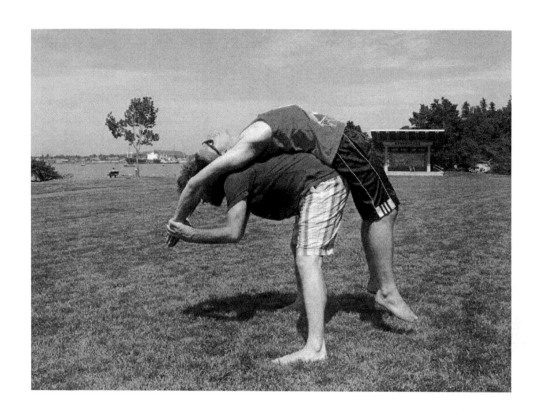

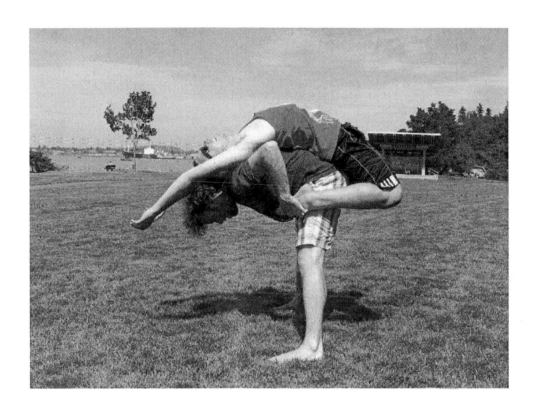

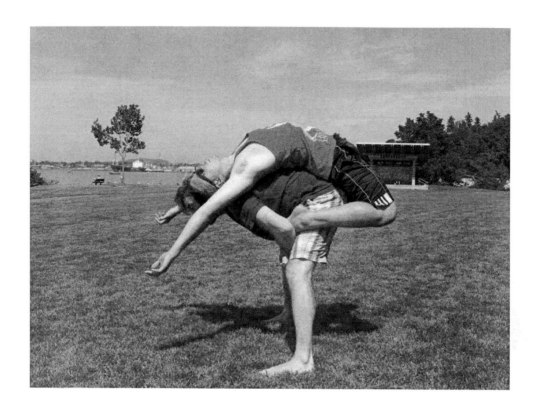

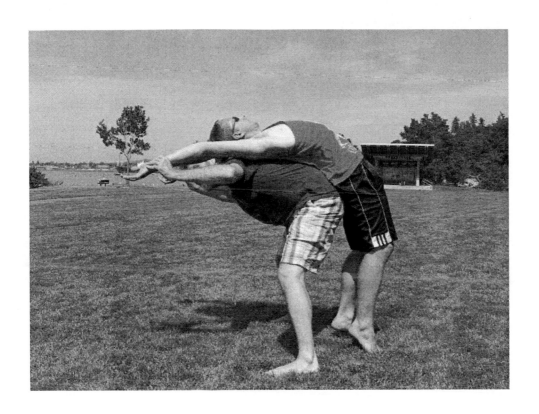

91-95. CLASSIC SEQUENCE #5: legagon (7)

91. legagon (7)

DESCR: Participants start in a circle, facing in towards the center. Raise right leg, take it further to the right, resting on neighbor's hip, making an 'M.C. Escher-style' staircase with the legs.
CAUTIONS:
CALLING: "Start in a circle facing toward the center, with hands to neighbor's shoulders. Now lift your right foot, and place it in the middle, then lift it and place it further off to the right, resting it on the right hip of the neighbor to your right. Make sure the heel is well past the edge of their thigh. Make any adjustments if you need to. Then take a breath or two here with the group. Tall spine, tall standing leg. Breathing nice and evenly."
NOTES:

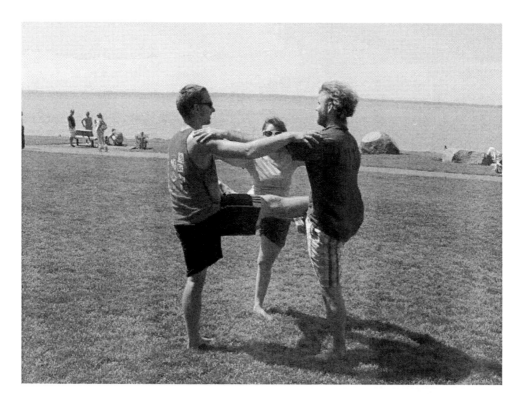

92. legagon huddle (7)

DESCR: Legagon legs, heads together in front, hands together in back.
CAUTIONS: Don't fall over. Don't push.
CALLING: "Start in legagon. Exhale, folding forward, bringing heads together in front and hands together in back. Hands can rest together with second neighbors' hands, or you can interlace the fingers. Breathing here several breaths. Inhale, coming back up to center. Exhale, rest."
NOTES:
VARIATIONS: Heads to neighbors' shoulders, instead of crown chakras, together in the middle.

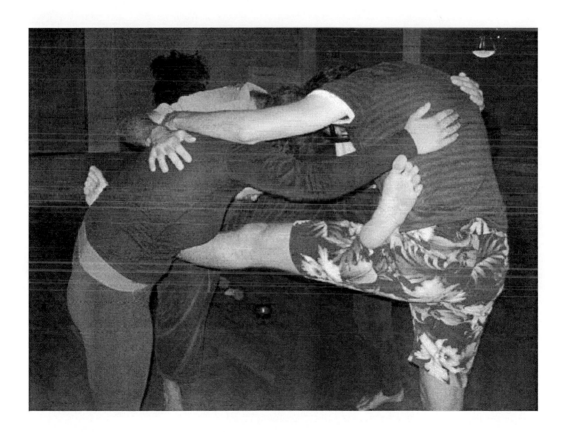

93. legagon leanback (8)

DESCR: Legagon legs, hands to neighbors' hands or wrists. Leaning gently back as far as is safe and comfortable.
CAUTIONS: Don't fall over. Don't pull too hard. Nice and slow, nice and steady. Stay centered. Evenly with the group.
CALLING: "Starting in legagon, you can bring your hands to neighbors' hands or wrists. Exhale, lean gently backwards, evenly with the group. Breathing here. Inhale, coming back up to center."
NOTES:

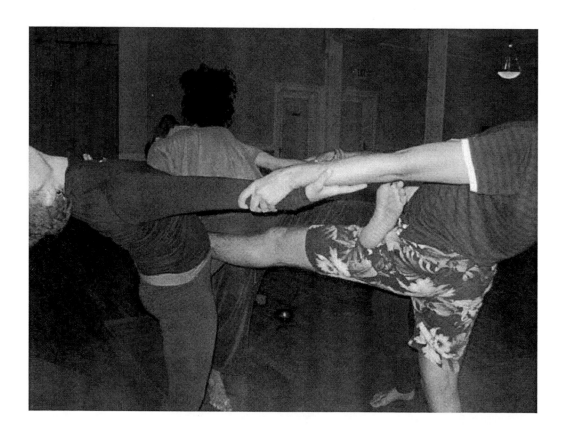

94. legagon cosmic spiral leanaway (7)

DESCR: Legagon legs. One hand together with the group in the middle, other hand opening out behind.
CAUTIONS: Don't fall over. Don't pull too hard.
CALLING: "Starting in legagon, place your right fingertips in the middle. Curl your hand together with the rest of the group. Inhale, open your left arm out behind you. Breathing here. Exhale, back to center. And we'll try it again on the other side."
NOTES:

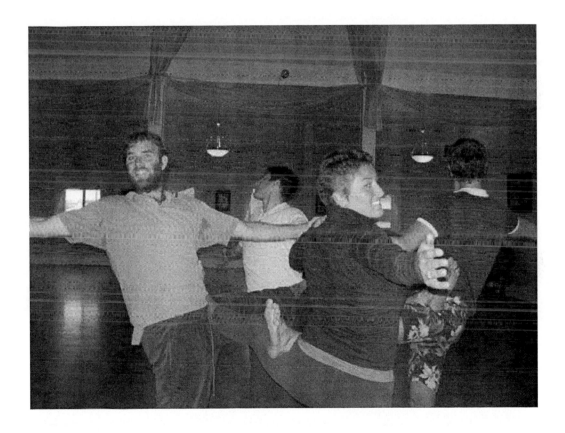

95. legagon hand-to-foot twist (7)

DESCR: Twist. With legagon legs, one hand reaches behind the back to grab neighbor's foot, other hand reaches across to opposite side to neighbor's shoulder.
CAUTIONS: Keep spine straight during twist. Don't sacrifice the integrity of the spine in an effort to twist or to grab the foot. Don't fall over. Don't pull too hard.
CALLING: "Starting in legagon, if your left foot is resting on neighbor's hip, take your right hand, reach around behind your back to find your neighbor's foot, take your left hand off to the right to find your neighbor's shoulder. Inhale, lengthen and straighten your spine. Exhale, twist to the right, looking over your right shoulder. Inhale back to center. Exhale, rest. Release."
NOTES:
SLANG NAMES: "legagon spinal twist A," "legagon foot twist."

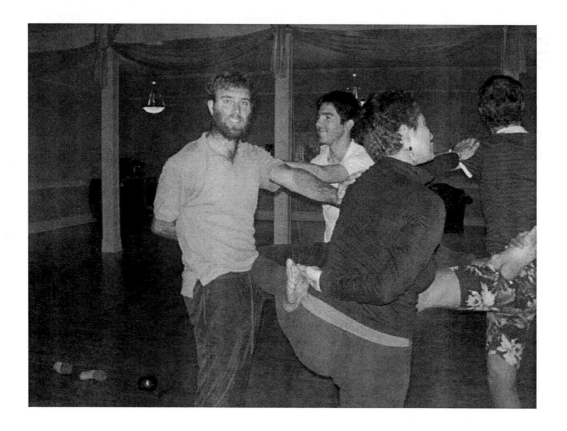

96. legagon hand-to-hand twist (8)

DESCR: Twist. With legagon legs, one hand reaches behind the back, second hand reaches across in the opposite direction to neighbor's hand.
CAUTIONS: Keep spine straight during twist. Don't sacrifice the integrity of the spine in an effort to twist or connect hands. Don't fall over. Don't pull too hard.
CALLING: "Starting in legagon, if your right foot is resting on your neighbor's hip, take your right hand behind your back, bending your right elbow. Now take your left hand, and reach off to your right, to find and grab the right hand of your neighbor to the right (which is sticking out from behind their back, waiting for you to grab ahold of it). Inhale, lengthen and straighten your spine. Exhale, twist and look to the right, looking over your right shoulder. Inhale, come back to center. Exhale, rest, releasing the hands and arms. If you need to come out, find neighbor's hands, bend both knees and come back down. Otherwise, continue on to the next pose."
NOTES:
SLANG NAMES: "legagon spinal twist B," "legagon hand twist," "legagon footless twist."

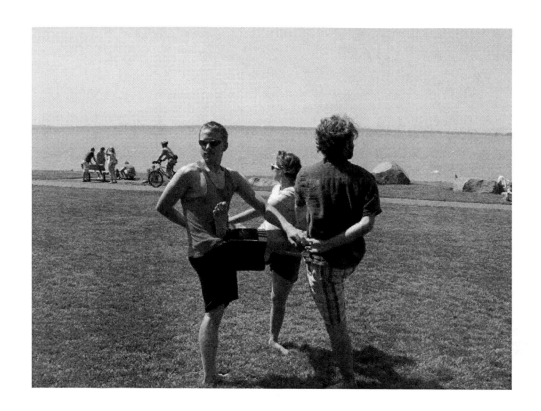

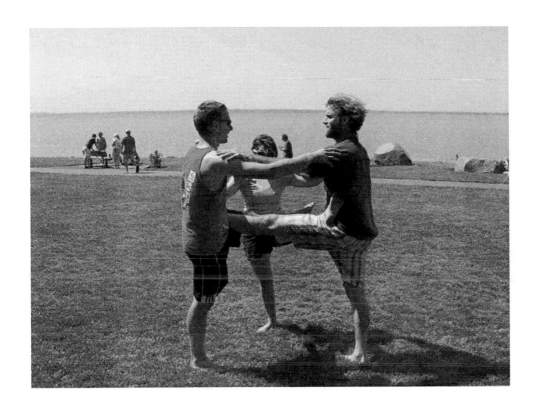

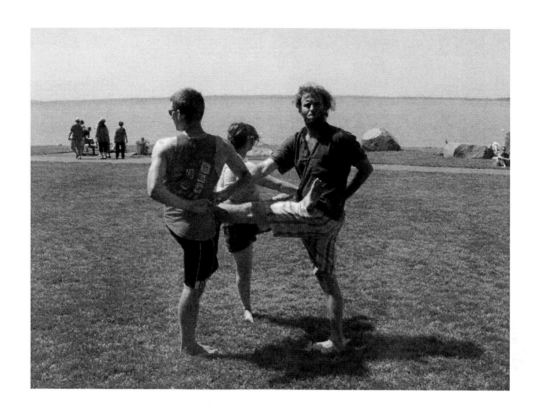

97. supported legagon (7)
DESCR: Inner layer in legagon, outer layer with hands gently resting on the backs of the hearts.
CALLING: "If you're in legagon, exhale forward, bringing heads together in the front and hands together in the back. If you're outside supporting, gently interlace hands with second neighbors and then place these shared hands on the backs of the hearts of your neighbors, on top of the legagon hands. Breathing here."
NOTES:
SLANG NAMES: "Loving legagon extended family."

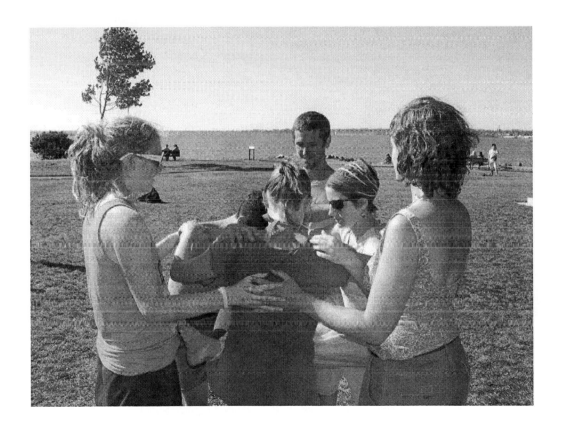

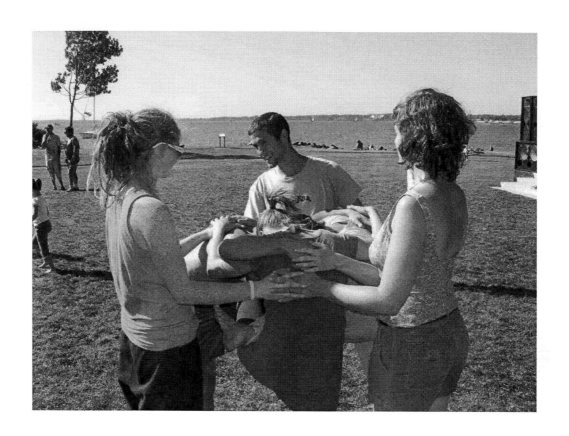

98-101. CLASSIC SEQUENCE #6: sloth family portrait (8)

98. sloth family portrait (8)

DESCR: Participants start in legagon. With legagon legs, forehead or cheek rests on neighbor's thigh, arms dangling down. If right leg is lifted to neighbor's hip, exhale forehead or cheek down to neighbor's thigh on your left.
CAUTIONS:
CALLING: "Start in legagon. Inhale lengthen, tall spine, tall standing leg. Exhale forward, and off to the side, away from your own raised leg, resting your forehead or cheek on neighbor's thigh, letting your arms dangle straight down. Breathing here. Continue to loving sloth family portrait, ambitious sloth family portrait, or inhale back up to center. Exhale, rest."
NOTES:

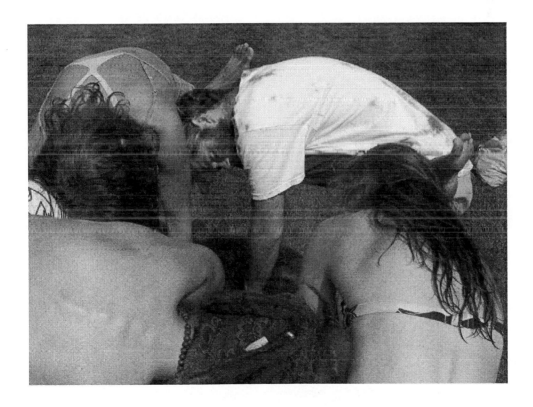

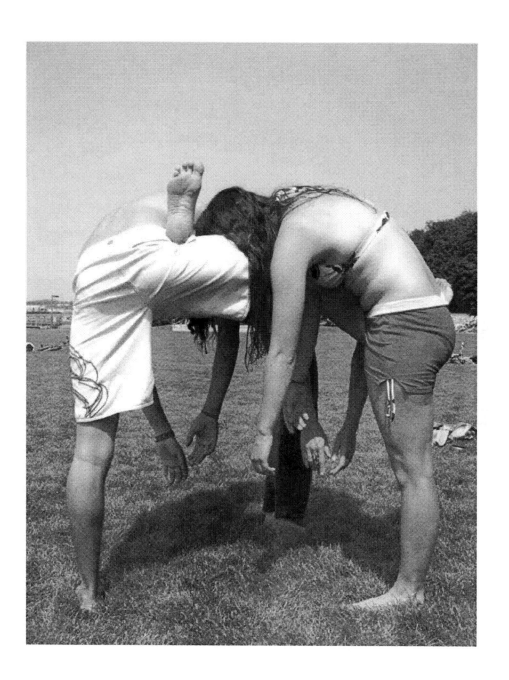

99. loving sloth family portrait (8)

DESCR: Same as sloth family portrait, but with all bottom (outside) hands together in the middle down below, all top (inside) hands to neighbor's cheek, head, neck, shoulder or back of heart.
CAUTIONS:
CALLING: "Start in sloth family portrait or ambitious sloth family portrait. Take bottom (outside) hand to back of neighbor's heart. Rest. Breathing here. Then continue to sloths play peek-a-boo, or inhale back up. Exhale, rest."
NOTES:
VARIATIONS: Bottom (outside) hands dangling down.

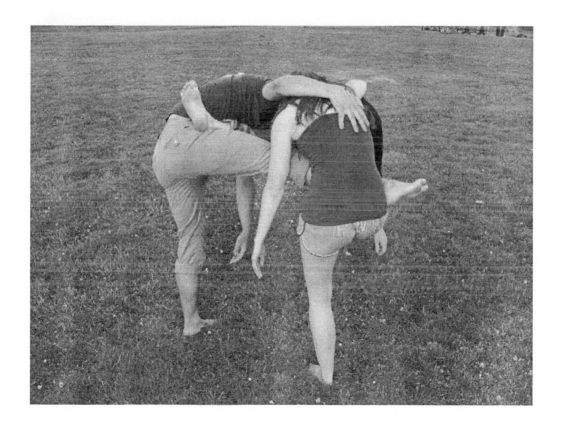

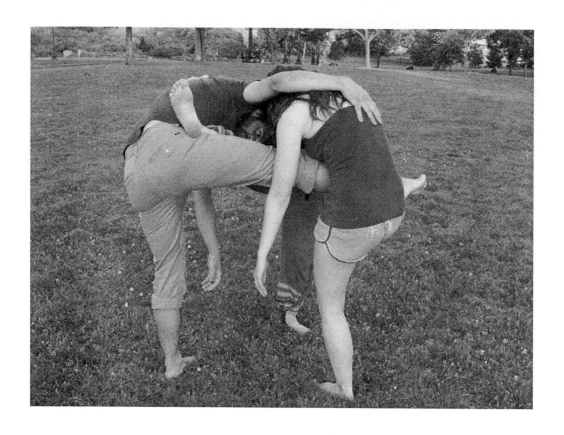

100. ambitious sloth family portrait (8)

DESCR: Same as sloth family portrait, but instead of both arms dangling down, everyone in the group puts one hand together in the middle on the bottom and one hand together in the middle on top.
CAUTIONS:
CALLING: "Start in sloth family portrait. Exhale, bottom (outside) hand to the middle, find the other right hands. Inhale, top (inside) hand to the top, finding all the other left hands. Breathing several breaths here. Continue on to loving sloth family portrait, sloths play peek-a-boo, or inhale back up to legagon. Exhale, rest."
NOTES:

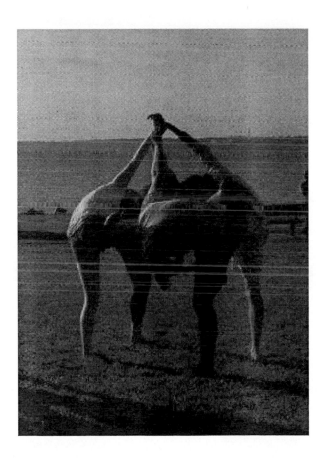

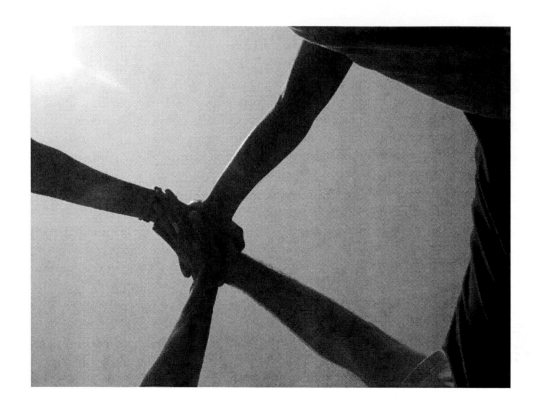

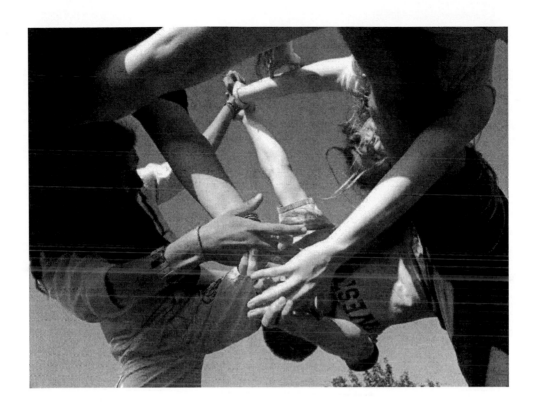

101. sloths play peek-a-boo (9)

DESCR: From ambitious sloth family portrait, heads go back and forth between resting on neighbor's thigh to looking at neighboring heads from underneath neighbor's leg.
CAUTIONS:
CALLING: "Start in ambitious sloth family portrait. Inhale, slightly lift head up off neighbor's leg. Exhale, duck head back around second neighbor's foot, taking head underneath neighbor's leg to look at your fellow peek-a-boo playing sloths. Smile. Breathing here. Inhale back up."
NOTES:

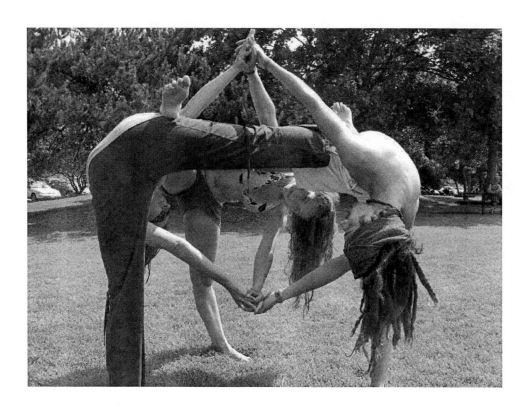

102. handstand pillars (8)

DESCR: Inner circle stands in Tadasana facing outward, handstands come up one at a time around the circle. Handstanders then come back down in the same 'domino' ('around-the-clock') around-the-circle fashion.

CAUTIONS: Agree on the order of coming up and coming down. Go slowly. Go in order. Keep the same order coming back down as you used going up, ie, whoever went up first, comes down first. Whoever went up second, comes down second, and so on. When coming down, take the legs back down to the outside of the circle. Do not roll forward to come out of your handstand. If more than one person does this, you will collide while on your necks!

CALLING: "Those on the inner circle stand, facing outward, ready to receive those who will be coming up into handstand. Once the order is clear… First handstander comes up, catch. Steady. Second handstander up, catch. Steady. Third handstander up, catch. Steady. And so on. First handstander back down. Steady. Second handstander back down. Steady. Third handstander back down. And so on."

NOTES:

VARIATIONS: Using core strength, all handstanders can take one leg down at the same time. Then repeat with the other leg. People in the inner circle can hold one leg apiece of two different handstanders' legs.

SLANG NAMES: "Handstand forest," "hands up, hands down."

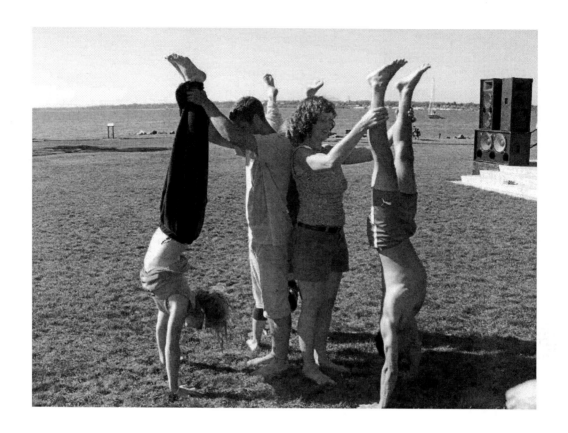

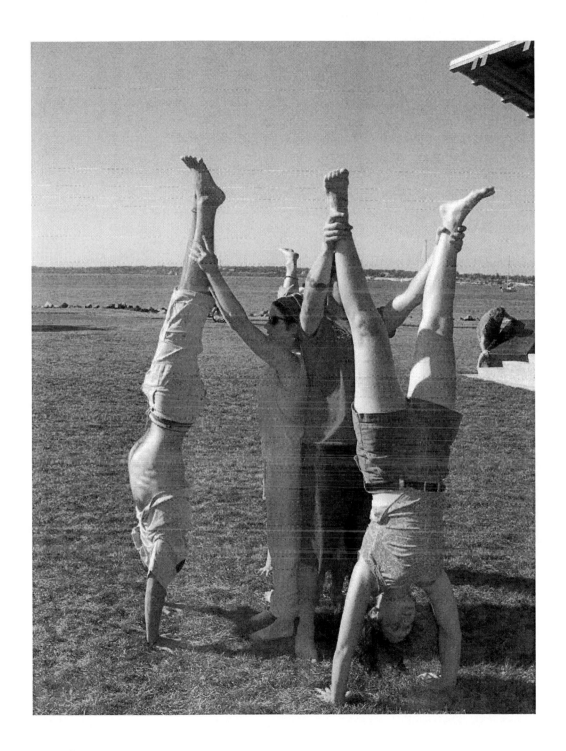

103. lumberjack free-hang (9)

DESCR: One person stands facing another. Second person does a handstand toward the first. First person grabs second person's ankles, slowly turns around. Second person bends their knees, draping their feet over first person's shoulders. First person lowers down, towards horse stance, weight low, leaning forward. With a very firm grip around second person's shins, first person can lean forward, lifting second person off the ground.

CAUTIONS: Do not lift someone who is more than 25 pounds heavier than you are. Practice and get comfortable with the mechanics of lifting with pose #90, standing back-to-back lift, before attempting this lift. Very important for the first person to keep their weight very low and very forward, or both people will be pulled to the ground backwards, in a very awkward and potentially harmful way for the first person's back and the second person's spine and neck. Lock arms firmly around shins. Strong grip.

NOTES:

VARIATIONS: Forward-facing version, with the free-hanger hanging off the front instead of the back.

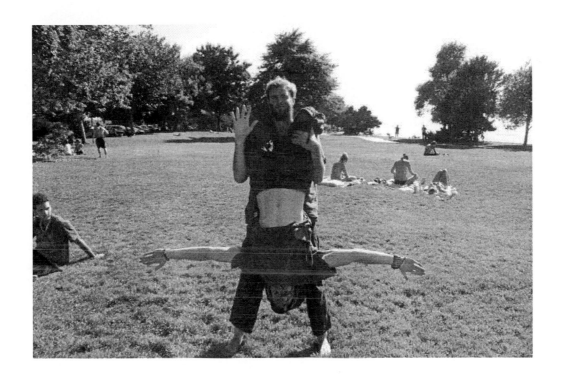

104. lumberjack chiropractor (9)

DESCR: One person stands facing another. Second person does a handstand toward the first. First person grabs second person's ankles, slowly turns around. Second person bends their knees, draping their feet over first person's shoulders. First person lowers down, towards horse stance, weight low, leaning forward. With a very firm grip around second person's shins, first person can lean forward, lifting second person off the ground. Second person relaxes completely, hanging freely, arms out to the sides. First person can lean forward, bringing their glutes and sacrum to press into the back of the second person.

CAUTIONS: Do not lift someone who is more than 25 pounds heavier than you are. Practice and get comfortable with the mechanics of lifting with pose #90, standing back-to-back lift, before attempting this lift. Exercise extreme caution. Have extreme fun.

NOTES: There is a 'sweet spot' where the backs of the bent knees of the person in free-hang fit snugly onto the shoulders of the lumberjack. By adjusting the height of the free-hanger, and then bending forward, the lumberjack can work their way down the back of the free-hanger, one vertebra at a time. Adjust height. Fold. Adjust height. Fold. And so on, down the spine.

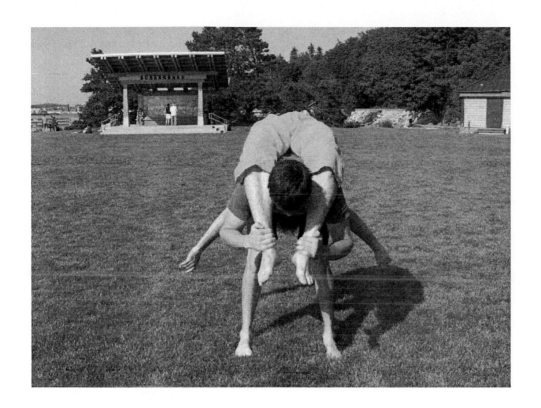

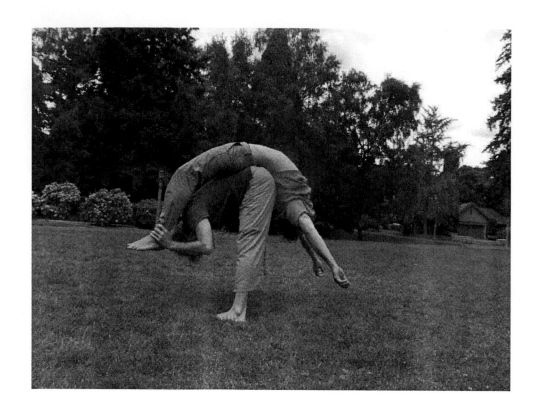

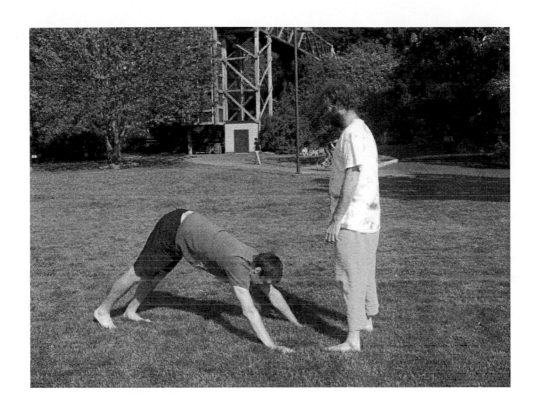

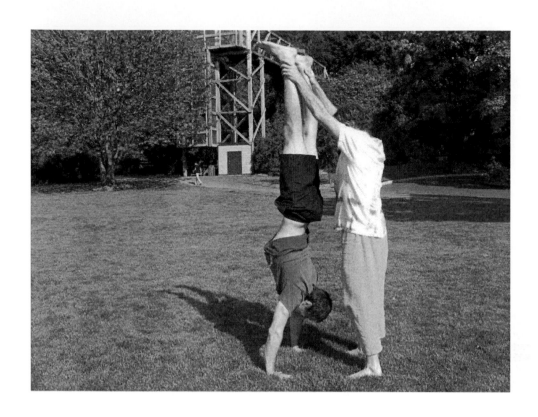

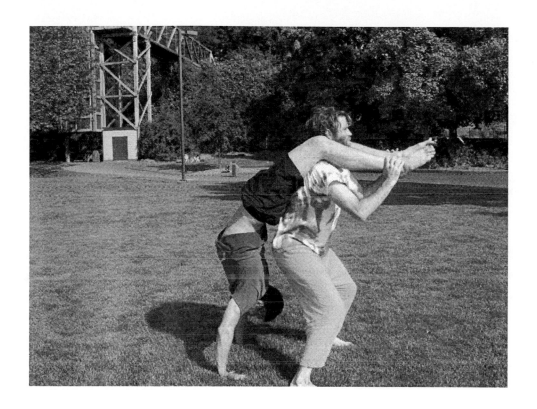

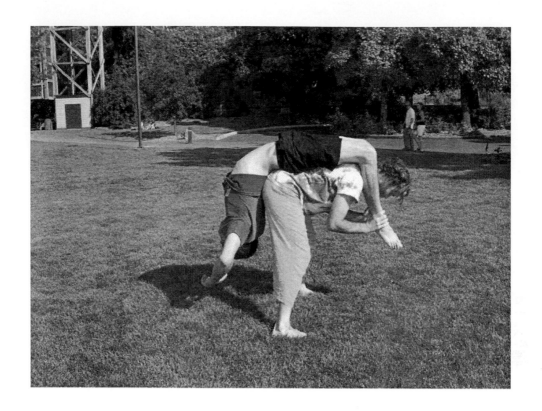

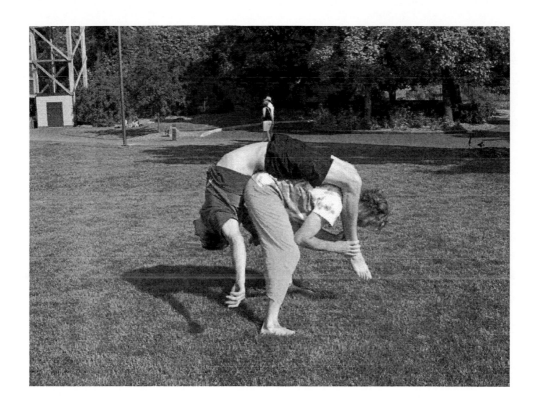

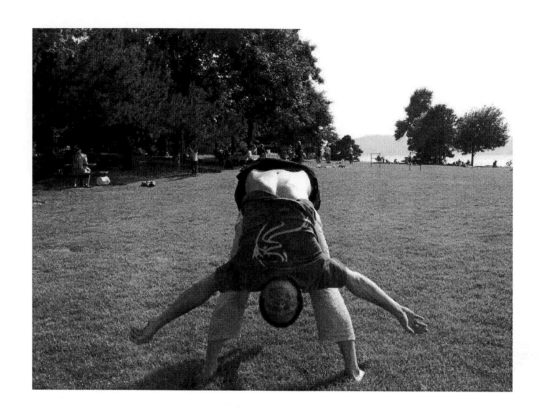

105. lumberjack ankle grab (9)

DESCR: One person stands facing another. Second person does a handstand toward the first. First person grabs second person's ankles, slowly turns around. Second person bends their knees, draping their feet over first person's shoulders. First person lowers down, towards horse stance, weight low, leaning forward. With a very firm grip around second person's shins, first person can lean forward, lifting second person off the ground. Second person, once they feel safe, can slowly reach for first person's ankles.

CAUTIONS: Do not lift someone who is more than 25 pounds heavier than you are. Practice and get comfortable with the mechanics of lifting with pose #90, standing back-to-back lift, before attempting this lift. Very important for the first person lifting the second to keep their center of gravity very low and lean strongly forward, or it's possible that both people will be pulled over backwards to the ground, in a very awkward way for the first person's back and the second person's spine and neck. Lock arms firmly around shins. Strong grip. Communicate clearly. Go slowly.

NOTES:

VARIATIONS: Forward-facing version, with the free-hanger hanging off the front instead of the back. If the liftee is extremely flexible, the lifter (lumberjack) can gently lean forward as in lumberjack chiropractor, while the liftee holds onto the ankles. This is very intense. Exercise extreme caution. Have extreme fun.

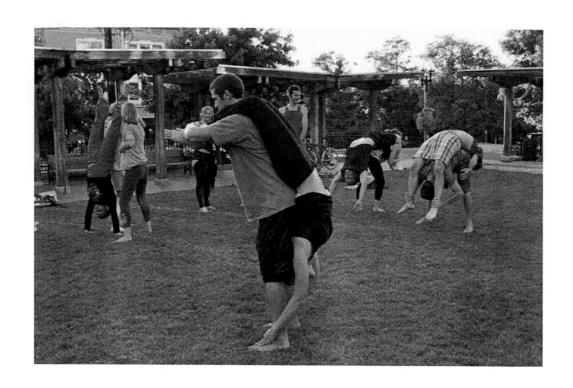

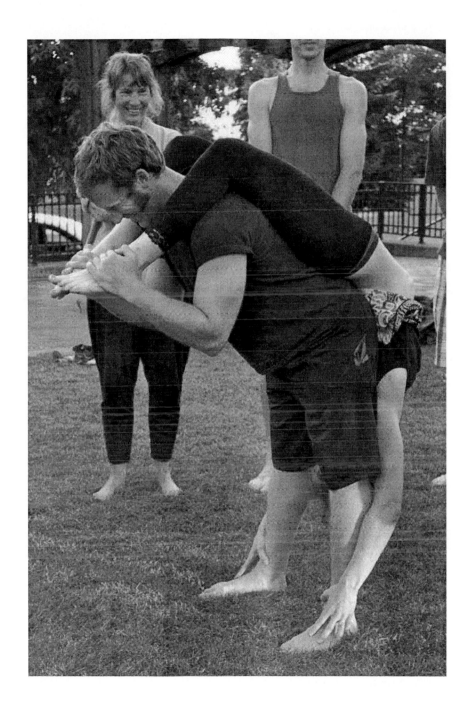

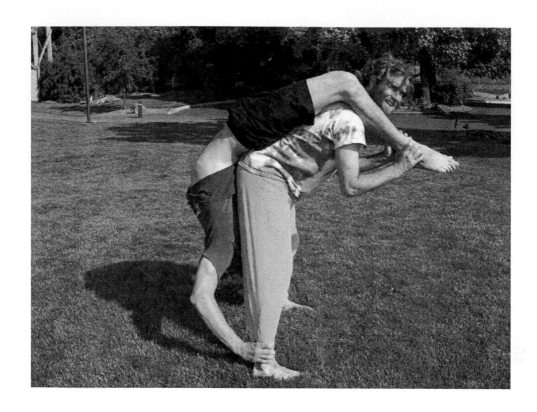

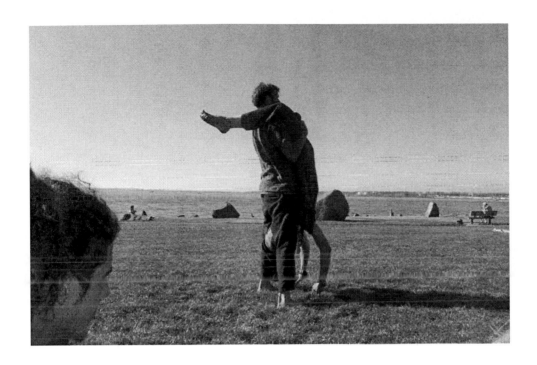

106. humaneering (partner climb-around) (9)

DESCR: One person, 'the climber,' climbs around another person 'the climbee,' in a vertical ellipse one or more times without touching the ground. To start, partners stand facing one another. First person, 'the climbee,' lifts up second person, 'the climber,' by the thighs, fireman carry style, then lifts them higher up onto one shoulder. Then, gently, mindfully, lets them down the backside, head-first, like the world's most precious sack of potatoes. Then, takes the near leg (next to the head) over to the other side of their head, so one leg is now on either side, head poking up through the middle. Then, one leg at a time, switch the arms so that instead of reaching around the outside of the legs to the top of the legs, the arms are now sticking up on the inside of the legs, hands on top of the heels. At this point, the 'climber's legs are around the torso of the first person, underneath the first person's arms. The second person's head is looking forward through the first person's legs. With the sacrum underneath the climber's pelvis, practice pressing down on the climber's heels and moving around from side-to-side in this locked and solid position. This is known as 'base camp.' From here the climbing begins. The climbee locks one arm around one leg of the climber. The climber, just like a rock climber would, swings their other leg (the free leg) around and underneath the first person's legs and out front, bracing the leg over the first person's leg on the same side. Now the two grab hands at an opposite diagonal. Grab onto the other hand as well. Hanging onto the arms, with one leg braced around the climbee, the climber works their second leg around to the front by bending the knee and sneaking underneath and then bringing the leg up on top of the climbee's second leg. With both hands diagonally crossed, with both legs braced over the second person, they can now pull together to lift the climber up to the torso of the climbee, with legs wrapped around back (as if they were lovers). Now repeat, climbing over the other shoulder, or come down and rest. See how many times you can go around, without touching the ground. I believe our record is eight times. Send us video if you break the record.
CAUTIONS: Do not lift someone who is more than 25 pounds heavier than you are. Practice and get comfortable with the mechanics of lifting with pose #90, standing back-to-back lift, before attempting this lift. Don't hurt yourself trying to break the record. For most people, once or twice is plenty.
NOTES: Communicate clearly. Go slowly.
VARIATIONS: You tell us.

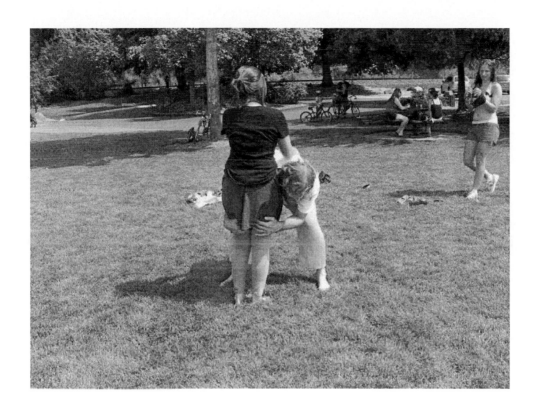

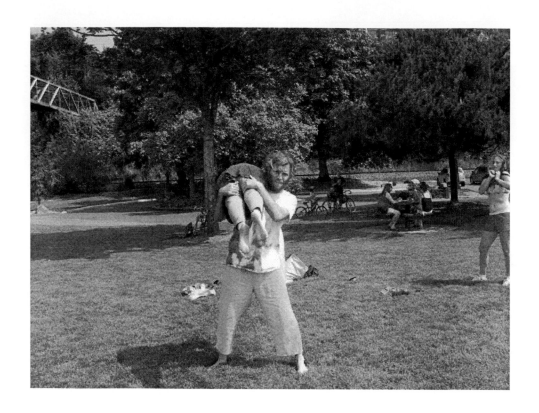

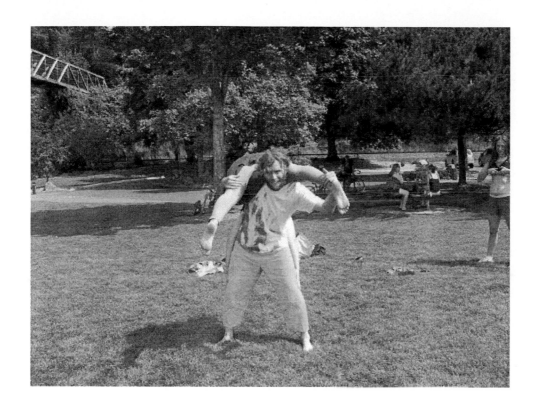

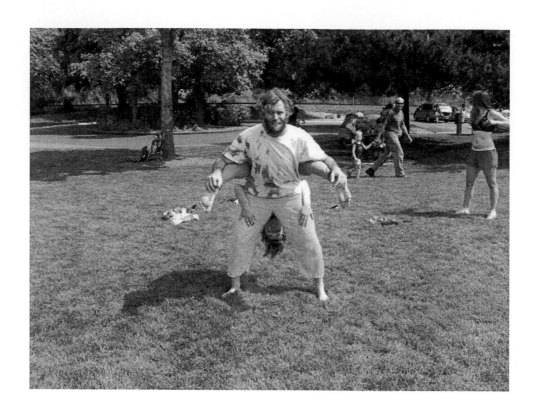

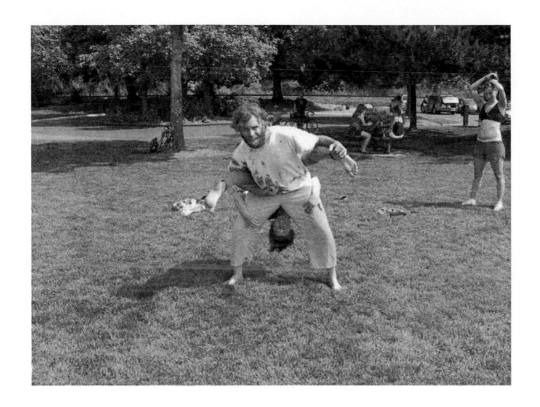

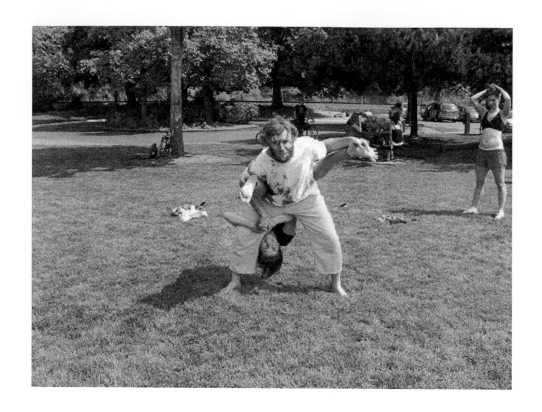

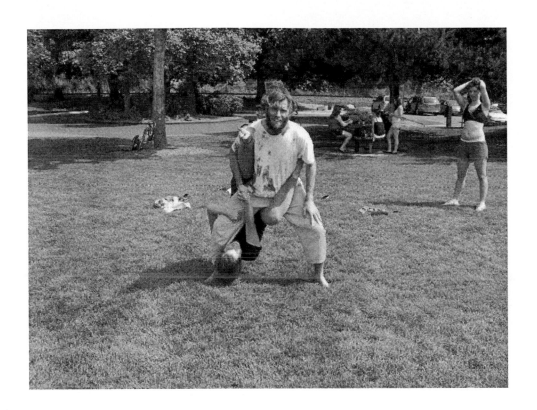

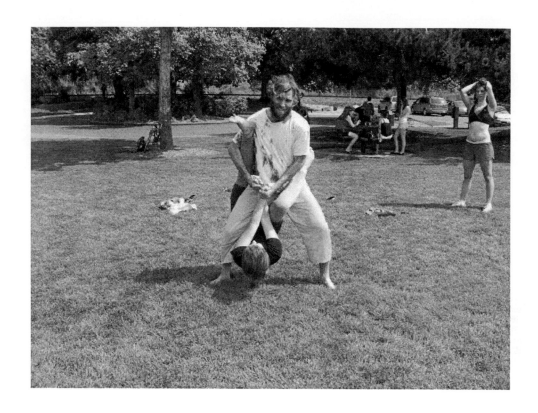

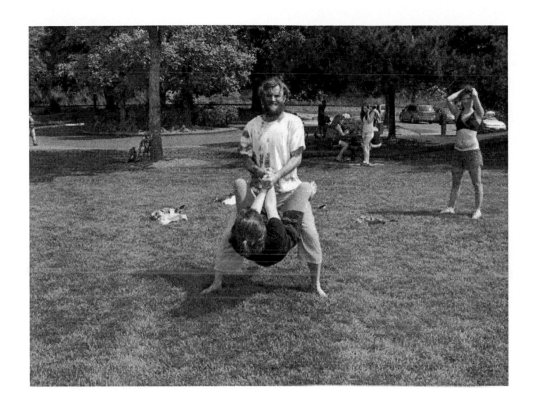

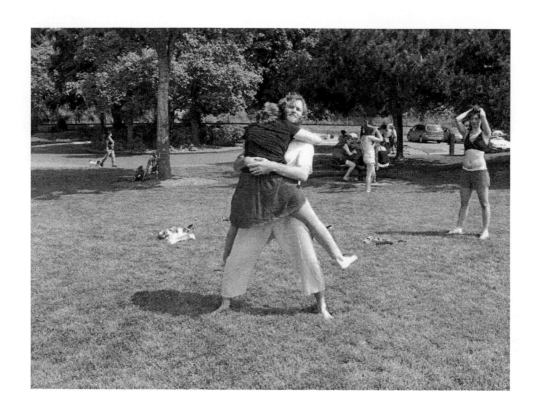

107. diamond dogs with partial (1-person) levitation (9)

DESCR: Participants start on all fours, facing one another backwards, ready to come up into downward-facing dog.
CAUTIONS: Do not lift someone who is more than 25 pounds heavier than you are.
CALLING: "Exhale, curl the toes and come into down dog. Inhale, lift your right foot, finding partner's right foot (this should be a diagonal line across and between your two bodies). Pressing your legs against one another, raising the feet up to the top together, making a nice diamond shape with your legs. Once both partners are up, decide who is going to lift their second leg up, and who is going to keep one leg on the ground. To provide more support, the person who is going to keep one leg on the ground can re-adjust so their foot is under the ankle or bottom of the shin of the person who is going to lift one leg up even higher. Once both feet are up off the ground, resting on only one foot of the partner, breathe here for a few breaths. Then exhale, bring one foot back down. Try the other foot. Breathe a few breaths. Bring one foot down. Exhale, both partners bring the second foot down at the same time. Both partners, inhale, bend both knees, coming to the ground. Exhale, sink into child's pose. Switch roles and repeat."
NOTES:
VARIATIONS: The person lifting a second leg into the air can stack the second foot on top of the first or keep raising that leg to vertical in a handstand variation.
RELATED POSES: See also, pose #56, diamond dogs.

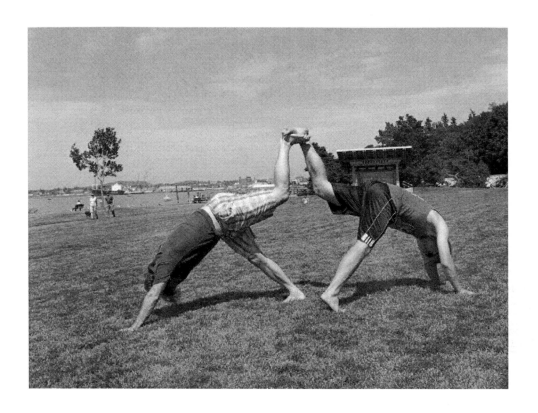

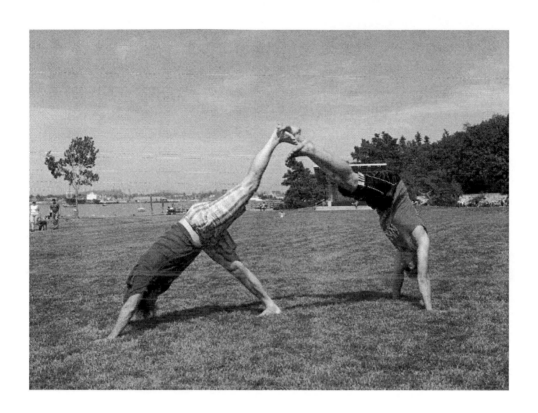

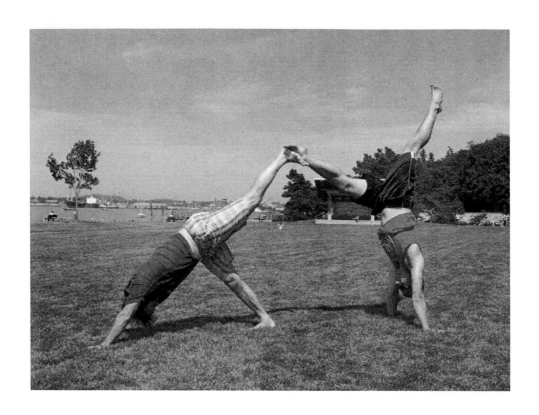

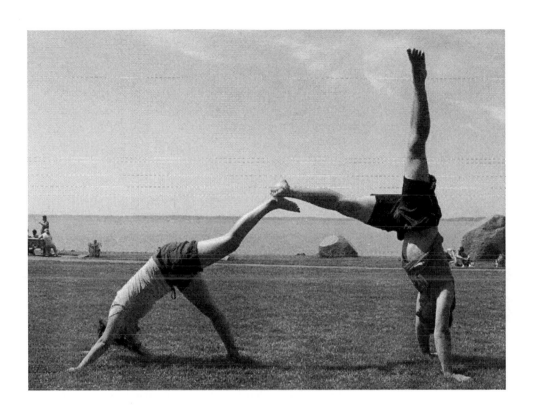

108. davinci's counterbalance (9)

DESCR: Two suspended splits counterbalances, back-to-back in such a way that those leaning back can rest their heads on one another's shoulders. One person crouches all the way down to the ground. Second person stands behind the first, with their knees bent and together. First person leans back until their shoulders are resting on the second person's knees, lifts their arms straight up overhead and clasps their hands behind the person's waist. Second person leans back. Once a point of balance is reached, the first person can carefully (one leg at a time) lift their legs up so the second person can grab one, and then both, of the first person's heels. The first person can then slowly, carefully lower one leg at a time, out straight and long, with toes pointed. The people leaning back can have their heads resting on one another's shoulders and their free arm raised behind them. Once you've done both legs, slowly bend the knees and come down one leg at a time. Second person help lift them up. First person unclasp the hands. Voilá!
CAUTIONS: Do not lift someone who is more than 25 pounds heavier than you are. Practice this and get comfortable with this as a partner exercise with plenty of space around, before attempting to bring two pairs together into davinci's counterbalance. Move slowly and carefully. Stay leaning back. Only move one leg at a time.
NOTES: The person who will be leaning back and lifting the other person off the ground can scoot forward or back to adjust the position of their knees in the shoulders of the person who will be lifted. This is helpful when working with people of different heights.
VARIATIONS: You tell us.

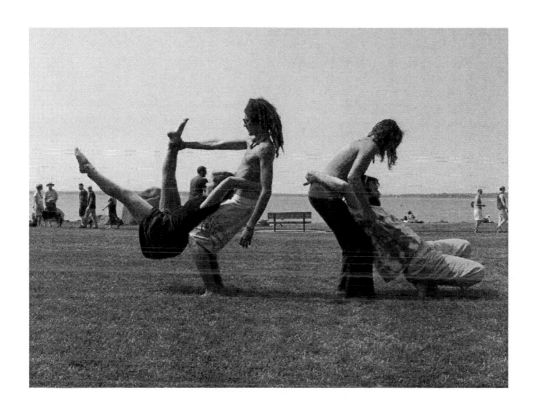

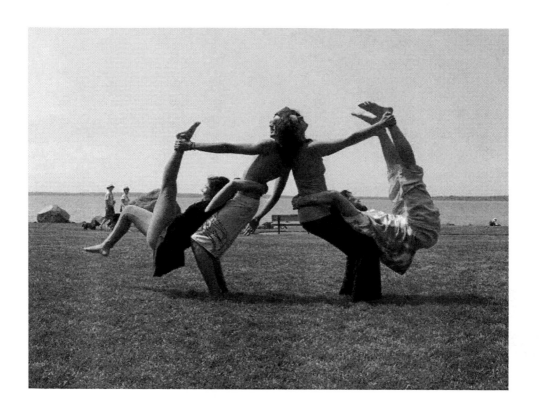

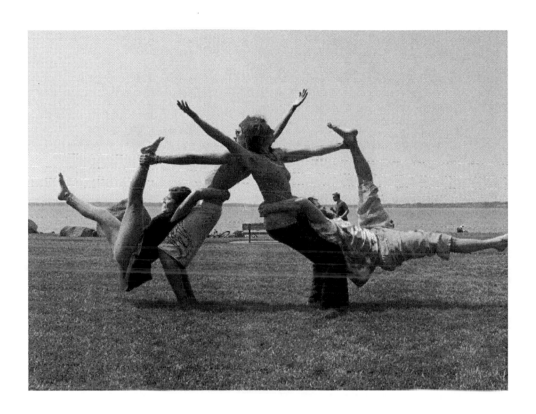

NOTES, REFLECTIONS, AND COMMENTARY

A full treatment of all the various topics related to the study of community yoga lies outside the scope of this book. This book is intended as an introduction and general guide to the concept of community-focused yoga poses, and as a manual or handbook that presents a specific style or system or set of poses, so that people can start practicing. A more exhaustive series of guidebooks, notes, reflections, and commentary on the poses, the project, community yoga practice, and related topics is forthcoming, but we have included here are a few very general notes and answers to a few common questions to help get you started.

Who can practice Kaleidoscope?
Everyone.

Where can you practice Kaleidoscope?
Anywhere.

Why 108 poses?
Short answer: 108 is a very auspicious number with many mathematical and spiritual significances.

What qualities are helpful for practicing Kaleidoscope?

openness	mindfulness
humility	safety
respect	patience
reflection	study
inclusivity	diversity
harmony	order
trust	communication
clarity	calm
sensitivity	strength
focus	balance
flexibility	

What's the biggest number of people you've ever had in one shape?
Well, (as a planet), let's find out...

GENERAL RECOMMENDATIONS

Have fun.
Don't try too hard.
Be mindful.
Be respectful.
Connect.
Listen.
Safety first.
Be patient and supportive of yourself and others.
Smile.
Bow.
Breathe.
If something is unclear, ask.
If something feels uncomfortable, back off or ease out of it. If something looks like it would be uncomfortable for you, don't do it. You can always be a witness or try a pose another time.
Advise the facilitator and the group of any special modifications or needs.
A little laugh and a friendly smile can go a long way.

NOTES ON BEGINNING AND CLOSING A SESSION

Always start each session with an intention and acknowledgment of the activity and the group at hand. Sharing some silence, holding hands, breathing together, chanting together and sharing names are good ways to do this. In extremely large groups, or in the case of brief demonstrations with larger groups, where there is a limited time allotted and sharing every single person's name would require more time than is practical, a moment of silence or prayer may suffice, but it is always important to acknowledge the group and its members and the intention of the time together.

For example, the facilitator might say, "Take a look around, and just notice and feel the group." Or… "Maybe notice your neighbor on either side." It's good to be here with this group, the…" Or…

"Welcome to Kaleidoscope. Welcome to this community yoga session here at Earth Day 2012 in Portland, Oregon. Thank you so much for coming and sharing." Etc, etc. Some sort of welcome and gratitude and acknowledgment of the moment and the group at hand is always appropriate.

Similarly for closing, some sort of acknowledgment of the close of the session is always recommended, even if people stay afterwards or hang out after the official closing. Shavasana, seated or standing heart circle, a chime, chanting, silence, prayer, a bow, or some combination is always appropriate.

NOTES ON THE PRACTICE OF A NAME CIRCLE

In general, it is always best to do a name circle. It's a good way to introduce people to one another, and to announce and acknowledge who is present. It is a good practice, even if everyone already knows everyone else's name. There is an element of ritual and power and strength and solidarity to it. It is also a way of officially saying, we are here now and we are starting now.

Let us reflect briefly a little further on the significance of this practice.

It is also (and this is very important) a way of signaling, right from the start, that everyone is included, that everyone gets a turn, and that we rotate through things as a group.

Everyone is an equal participant.

Even if only briefly, every single person has a place and a voice within the circle.

And, again, in turns, even if only briefly, everyone in the circle is silent, and is practicing listening to the other members of the group, as a whole, and to each one individually. This is very important.

As a facilitator, taking the time to do a name circle signals to the group that you acknowledge every person in the circle, and that everyone is important. If anyone joins the circle after the session has started, have that person share their name as a way of acknowledging their addition to the group.

This simple, but profound act of listening and acknowledging will lead to a smoother session and more harmonious energy within the group.

NOTES ON THE ROLE OF THE FACILITATOR

The facilitator has a very special role within a Kaleidoscope yoga community. The facilitator is the energetic anchor of the group. The role of the facilitator is to guide the group, to turn the tube of the Kaleidoscope, metaphorically speaking. The facilitator serves as the voice that organizes the shapes, and provides instruction for those who need it. It is the responsibility of the facilitator to make sure everyone is included, to keep everyone safe, to set the tempo and tone of the session, to keep the energy calm and harmonious, and to make sure that the energy is shared evenly within the group.

When people have ideas for new poses, new variations, or new sequences, it is also the role of the facilitator to help establish a sense of order and procedure for accepting and processing this input.

NOTES ON THE SELECTION OF A FACILITATOR

Many people who are enthusiastic or devoted or advanced students of yoga are not necessarily suitable choices for facilitation.

Not everyone has the temperament, interest, patience, or ability to be a facilitator. The facilitator must value the safety and progress of the group and of everyone in it, over their own ego or reputation, and genuinely want everyone in the group to grow and succeed.

Anyone can practice and enjoy Kaleidoscope, but it is very strongly recommended that anyone interested in guiding or leading a regular group of shared yoga practice seek out and receive training in the art of facilitating community yoga.

NOTES ON FACILITATION

Facilitating community yoga is an art form and an entire field of study unto itself. Facilitation is a skill, a process, and a journey. While it is outside the scope of this book to give a more in-depth treatment of the art of facilitation, we offer here a few notes and tips.

It is important to finish whatever pose or sequence you are working on. Always do both sides.

If you don't finish the pose or sequence you're working on and jump right to someone's new idea, just because they are enthusiastic, then you are signaling to the group that the sequence you were in the middle of was not important.

Furthermore, if you jump too quickly from one idea to the next, without patience and a sense of order, you may suddenly find that you have several subgroups doing lots of different things, on different timing, and that the group energy is scattered and off-track.

WITNESSING

Witnessing is an important practice, in Kaleidoscope, and in life in general.

Observing the forms, from many angles, from inside the shapes and out, can be a helpful study, and an illuminating practice. And it's enjoyable. A healthy balance of both "being in the shapes" and "being outside the shapes" is recommended for all participants, including those facilitating.

ADJUSTING THE NUMBERS
The facilitator and willing members of a group can alternate between "being in the shapes" and "being outside the shapes", in order to slightly adjust the numbers of a group to a desired number for the purpose of making a specific shape.

A NOTE ON THE LEVELS OF DIFFICULTY
The intention behind the practice of labeling individual poses with an approximate level of difficulty is simply to keep people safe. It's not a contest. It's not a point system. It's not a hierarchy. There's no moral judgment involved. And what one person may find challenging or delicate, another person may find simple and straightforward. And even the same person may find that the difficulty of a pose varies from day to day or over longer periods of time. It's simply an approximate framework designed to forewarn people which poses may need more warm-up, practice, balance, strength, or flexibility.

NOTES ON THE SHARING OF ENERGY
Sharing one's energy evenly with everyone in the community is one of the great joys and lessons and deeper truths of Kaleidoscope yoga practice, and of life in general. There is no way to over-emphasize this point.
When you shake up the pieces of a kaleidoscope, they fall where they fall, and they continue combining and recombining in every possible combination. The pieces don't decide that they only want to combine with certain other pieces. They don't have preferences. A willingness to partner and combine with anyone in the group is a sign of maturity within Kaleidoscope practice. Having said that, we are sensitive, vulnerable beings, and no one ever needs to feel pressure to do any pose they don't want to do, or to work with someone they feel uncomfortable with, or be in a pose that makes them uncomfortable. Over time, with care and mindfulness on the part of everyone, trust builds naturally with people who return to the shapes again and again.
During a jam, bringing the group back into one big circle for large group circle poses, even repeating the same pose several times in the same session, for the purpose of synchronizing the group, is recommended. It is a good way to integrate new members into the group, and for mature, well-practiced members of the group,

reviewing the fundamentals and deepening into the same poses over and over again is always good practice.

For safety reasons, or if someone is uncomfortable with a pose, anyone may always choose not to do a pose, (which is fine), but once a pose is offered to the group, it is extremely important that the facilitator rotate the option of any pose offered to the group to every member of the group. It is also important to follow through and finish any sequence one starts and do both sides of every pose. Enthusiasm for a new pose idea or excitement over a request is not sufficient reason to not rotate evenly through the group or do both sides.

Slow, systematic rotation keeps the energy evenly distributed and harmonious, and keeps the group energy from getting distracted, scattered, fragmented, diffuse, or unsafe.

NOTES ON SAFETY AND GROUP POSES
It is very important to take extra precautions to see to it that everyone is safe, especially when participants are sharing weight. Because of the interconnected nature of community yoga shapes, this is even more important than usual. When an individual comes down out of a pose, or falls off balance, or falls down, with enough space, the person can respond or recover or land or roll as they see fit. With group poses, however, this freedom of movement and space can be limited by the other people in the pose. In legagon and community acro shapes, for example, falling out of balance can actually pull several people out of balance, with little or no room to adapt or adjust. Caution and mindfulness are always encouraged. Thankfully, there is an opportunity for more balance and support with community yoga poses as well.

ON MULTIPLE FACILITATORS OR A FACILITATOR AND ASSISTANTS
It is also possible to have multiple people taking turns facilitating or co-facilitating, or to have a teacher and assistants. This was the original vision, a caller, and several assistants. Practice of this style and research into it, is ongoing.

MATHEMATICS AND SACRED GEOMETRY
Mathematics and sacred geometry is an enormous field of study, and the application of sacred geometry to collective human yoga is an even larger, richer

field of study. For those interested, we recommend a deeper study of mathematics and sacred geometry.

A NOTE ON MOSAICS
Within the context of Kaleidoscope Community Yoga, a 'mosaic' refers to putting several group yoga shapes together in the form of a pattern. To give one of the simplest examples, several grass-in-the-wind hexagons can be placed next to one another in a honeycomb pattern. This would be called a 'grass-in-the-wind hexagon mosaic.' A full treatment of the study of mosaics as it applies to shared community yoga practice is forthcoming. This book is a presentation of some of the most basic building blocks or puzzle pieces that can be made by combining yoga shapes together. But it is only the beginning. Amazing new layers of subtlety and interconnection are possible when these basic shapes are combined into even larger, layered, more complicated shapes, designs, and mosaics.

HISTORY, ORIGINS, INFLUENCES, VISIONS AND MYTHOLOGY

HISTORY: THE STORY OF KALEIDOSCOPE IN THE MAKING

What is the history of Kaleidoscope Community Yoga and of the Kaleidoscope Community Yoga project?

What a messy question. It is my least favorite.

The way it usually comes about is I start showing someone some group yoga poses and then at some point, they say something like, "Whoa, cool. Where did you get this? Where did you learn how to do this? Where does this come from?" An innocent, but loaded, misleading, and inevitably awkward question.

If I say that I invented it, I feel strange and shy and sheepish and awkward and proud and like I'm bragging about something I shouldn't be bragging about, all at the same time. If I try to defer, they want to know where I learned it or who I learned it from. To which I can only say, I didn't learn it from anyone or anywhere else, I learned it from me. From inside. I'm teaching it to other people. We are the source. I have learned many things from many people and practices (see the influences section) and have incorporated many things that we discovered as a group. Maybe one could say that I made many important discoveries, systematized it, compiled it, and organized it. There, that sounds a little better. But I also sort of invented it. With lots of help, of course.

Words and history, and the question of origins, are such a mess. Just look at the photos and practice with your friends. Everyone would be so much better off. Really.

Another version of the story (before I tell the one that people want to hear), that I often believe and would often like to tell people (but that not very many other people seem to find credible) goes something like this:

For me, Kaleidoscope Community Yoga is its own field of study, its own foundation, its own source, its own history, its own essence, its own spirit, its own energy, its own myth, its own being.

My soul is probably roughly 34 million years old, much of which time was probably spent as water, undersea creatures, rocks, herons, otters, caves, clouds, and in meditation.

The community yoga forms come through me from somewhere else, and I simply recognize them when they do. It's a combination of humanity, God, totem spirits, light, energy, pure forms, shared somatic intelligence, or whatever divine benevolence you believe in.

If you believe in all sorts of dimensions and parallel universes and altered states of consciousness and astral planes, then a little bit of people sharing group yoga forms is no stretch of the imagination. If you don't believe in all those things, well, then, I don't know what to tell you. Read further to the next explanation, and see if you can believe that. That's the best I can do.

On a pragmatic level, the shapes exist, and they do work, regardless of 'where they come from.'

From the dreamtime, or a surrealist perspective, or a vibrational, energetic, multidimensional, holographic perspective, the whole idea of a (linear) history is a very small, limited, misguided, misleading, messy, mental construct fraught with all sorts of problems. Trying to encapsulate a deeper energetic understanding of the true nature and width and breadth of the community yoga project and its possibilities into a linear history in words across a few pages is a bit like trying to pull a regular sized human T-shirt over a horse. And that metaphor is actually probably a vast understatement. And yet, having said that, some people insist on doing so. And for those people, I will do my best to sketch out, as honestly as I can, the answer that I think they are looking for and will be willing to believe, and happy to hear. But let it be repeated that this is not my truest, deepest sense or beliefs about the yoga project and its 'history.' It is merely some potentially interesting anecdotes arranged in a way that people can easily make sense out of.

Having said all that, the question doesn't seem to be going away. So, once and for all, at the insistence of other people, I will do my best to answer it in a way that seems to be what people are looking for. Hopefully it will provide a little bit of human interest and entertainment, if nothing else.

Here it goes... a hodgepodge of tall-tale, memory, trivia, anecdotes, mythology, autobiography and pseudo-journalism, for those who insist on some sort of history for the yoga project, despite all of my objections to the contrary, and my own disbelief in the validity, profundity, rationality, and possibility of such an enterprise.

The story of Kaleidoscope that many people seem to want to hear, (or to be able to believe), of my own autobiography and yoga journey (in this lifetime), and the intertwined history of Kaleidoscope, in a more or less linear fashion... and it goes something like this. The dates are a little fuzzy.

I grew up in Kennewick, Washington. At the confluence of the Columbia, Yakima, and Snake Rivers. Tumbleweeds, ridiculous heat, and a nuclear reactor. I have been reading my whole life, since I was like two. My mother was a reading teacher. I have always loved reference books of all kinds. Dictionaries, wildlife encyclopedias, bird books, field guides, anything and everything. I have also been swimming my whole life. Plenty of time outdoors as a kid. Birdwatching and fly-fishing. Lots of soccer. My father did all sorts of things, among them a lot of work at the local landfill. He also coached my soccer team and painted watercolors and hunted and fished and was generally a very unique and interesting human being, to say the least. He owned his own business for most of my childhood and adult life. My mother grew up in Port Huron, Michigan. My father grew up in Flint, Michigan.

I have always been obsessed with infinity and water.

In Kindergarten, I have a distinct memory of a project where we were supposed to take little cubes of graph paper and cut them out, and (if need be) tape them together to make rows that would illustrate counting. One cube, two cubes, three cubes, etc. My teacher, noticing my absorption, ended up just leaving me out in the hallway the rest of the day, making longer and longer taped-together rows of cubes, instead of having me do whatever else was planned for the day. I ended up taping together rows of more than a thousand cubes. It sounds now, as an adult, like a colossal waste of paper, and that I must be exaggerating or remembering incorrectly, but I don't think I am. Growing up, I was always being told I was gifted in math, but always seemed to prefer art and reading.

I took a B.A. degree in philosophy at Linfield College, in McMinnville, Oregon. I also took many language classes. My favorite philosophy classes were Eastern Philosophy and Postmodern. I read piles and piles and was absolutely fascinated by many feminist writers, structuralists, deconstructionists, postmodernists, poststructuralists, and postcolonialists. I also loved reading anything having to do with languages, systems, structure, and theory in general.

I lived abroad in Chile for a semester during my senior year in college. Learned Spanish. Travelled to the Amazon and Maccu Piccu. Lived in Sweden for several months. Learned Swedish. Returned to the United States and moved to Portland, Oregon.

I was working at Powell's books in Portland, Oregon. There was a Secret Santa gift exchange. The person I was to buy gifts for was a yoga teacher by the name of Jill Hummelstein, who had studied a lot of Iyengar yoga. I ended up taking her yoga classes. She was my first yoga teacher. That was how I started getting involved with yoga. I had never tried it and knew (at least in practice) nothing about it. I have been studying yoga for about eleven years now. Over the next eleven years, I would take every yoga class I could find from every yoga teacher, style, and studio I could find. Too many to list.

About six years in to my study of yoga, I took a teacher training, with Abby Staten, who owned a studio called (fittingly enough) Everybody's Yoga. She had trained in Viniyoga with Gary Kraftsow, in the lineage of T.K.V. Desikachar. It was also at some point around this time, that I legally changed my name to Logermund Nathamundi, (I was born John Kenneth Zillich, and grew up as a child with the name "J.K.") after stewing on it and meditating on it for about a year. Shortly thereafter, my yoga teacher said to me, "Did you know that there is a famous 10th century yogi scholar monk in the same lineage that you've been studying, named Nathamuni?" And I said, matter-of-factly, and I quote, "No."

About seven years in, I started teaching yoga.

About eight years in, I was doing a lot of thai massage at the time, I started teaching partner poses in my classes. I noticed that some students stopped coming to my classes because the partner poses made them uncomfortable, but the ones who did stay seemed to enjoy the partner poses and benefit from them immensely. After a while of practicing the same partner poses again and again, the regulars in my yoga classes actually seemed, it seems odd to put it this way, but I swear it's true, very familiar and almost sort of bored with them. I also began to notice a sort of choreography developing, or almost developing, or wanting to develop, as I watched the group do partner poses. I got so familiar with the partner poses, that I started looking through them and seeing the group shape that the partners were in, and noticing the negative spaces in between the students. Some of the more familiar and experienced students would also sometimes bump into one another and then smile, or intentionally try to reach across to the next pair over. And then I had the original Eureka moment: What if we make up a whole new activity of group yoga poses? The second thought revolution, immediately after the first: What if becomes as popular and normal as roller skates and salsa dancing or knitting or fishing or whatever people consider normal? The goal, the quest, the vision, of seeing how many people we could get doing this thing and to see how normal we could make it, was born. What was it? A social activity? A sport? A game? A hobby? A spiritual practice? All of the above? It also felt like we needed (or wanted) a name for this thing we were doing. After several weeks (or was it months?) still without a good name for this new activity, another Eureka came, the name: Kaleidoscope! That's it! That's what it's going to be called. That's what it *has* to be called. The theme, the metaphor. It's perfect. I raced to the Internet and did a search for Kaleidoscope Community Yoga. Nothing came up. Absolutely nothing. Not a single result. Perfect.

About nine years into my yoga career, I officially started the Kaleidoscope Community Yoga project as its own entity. Kaleidoscope Community Yoga was born in Bellingham, Washington. The first Kaleidoscope Community Yoga class was held in early 2010 at Presence Studio, run by Jenny Macke, in downtown Bellingham. It was open to the public, entirely group-pose based, and by donation.
It all snowballed from there. The rest was either downhill (synchronicity, magic, coincidence, flow, adventure) or uphill (hard work, transcription, study, labor, promotion, documentation, explanation, administration, organization.) or around the hill, or through the hill. But whichever way it rolled, up, down, all over the place, the community yoga ball has never stopped rolling. From that initial question and revelation, the rest has been history. The rest has been discovery and mapping, organization and administration, practice, play, exploration and inspiration.

About six months into the project, we had our first Kaleidoscope Crew, in the fall of 2010. The intention behind crew was to have a group of people who were more than just regulars, who wanted to help design and discuss the poses and the project, and organize and promote the project. A volunteer staff, basically. There were 4 people. It was myself, one of my best friends Brian Anderson, a tireless fan, supporter and servant of the project in the early days, another one of my best friends Alex Peregrina, who ended up taking an enormous amount of photographs for the project, perhaps more than any other single person, and Desirae Hill, who ended up being our graphic, web, and logo designer. We met at Café Bloom, an all organic, all vegan café in downtown Bellingham, run by Justin Bilancieri, that is sadly no longer there. Besides our first crew meetings, we also had our first level 2, or K2, jams in the back of Café Bloom. I think we were calling them 'jams' instead of 'classes' by then. If $9 came in as donations, we would give Justin $2 or $3. And, when the staff wasn't busy, we would show off our newest combinations and try to get them to join us. Hang out and eat healthy food. Those were the early days.

Even if we didn't know what it was or where it was headed, it grew. Our first special event was an artists' night, where local artists could draw these strange new yoga shapes we were making. At the time, it was our most well-attended, well-donated event to date. There were 18 people there. $84 came in. Which, at the time, was mind-blowing. And our first newspaper reporter. First outside media. A reporter from the Western Front, the Western Washington University newspaper. The art that was made was put onto my first business cards.

In a relatively short time, with an astonishing amount of hard work, the project grew with an astonishing amount of success. Particularly successful was combining community yoga with groups who were already in existence. Raw potlucks, healing centers, music shows, campus meditation groups, etc.

And, of course, besides the 'official' jams and classes, we always did a lot of yoga in between. Just hanging out in the park. On the beach. In people's living rooms and backyards.

Kaleidoscope Community Yoga began with an idea and a group of friends sharing yoga together. And, in many ways, it still is just that, a group of friends sharing yoga.

We just have more practice, more poses, more experience, (hopefully) more wisdom, and (hopefully) more humility. We also have a website, shirts, a book, lots of photos, some video. A few investors. And a lot more fans and friends. And literally more than 20 notebooks filled with drawings. To this day, as documentation, I draw, describe, and make notes on every single pose and combination we do, which is something I have done from day one.

At some point down the road, after having started the project, and after having posted some of our first photos and creating a Facebook fan page, I searched the internet again for Kaleidoscope Community Yoga... What?!? There was now a Kaleidoscope Yoga in Mexico. And sometime later, a Kaleidoscope Kids Yoga in Ohio. I panicked. Perhaps not the best response, but that was what I did, initially. A little while later, shortly after I visited my brother in South Carolina, a new studio named Kaleidoscope Yoga opened up in South Carolina. The 100th monkey effect plus the Internet. None of them seemed to be doing what we were doing, but other people had started calling their yoga studio or their project Kaleidoscope after we put ourselves on the Internet. A whole new series of questions about patenting, trademarking, franchising, etc. went racing through my mind.

Shortly after Café Bloom closed their doors, we moved the project from Presence Studio and Café Bloom to the Majestic. The first jam at The Majestic, with help from Alborz Monjazeb, was in January of 2011.

We continued to travel and teach and share and practice. Performances, classes, workshops, and demonstrations in Washington and Oregon. Music shows and circus shows. A community yoga dance piece, a combination yoga and massage workshop and other projects.

Also notable. While at a Sustainable Bellingham roving garden party stop at Danielle AhMalua's house, Jeff Westcott jokingly suggested that we should do a roving yoga party tour, which sounded to me like a fantastic idea. It became the Sustainable Bellingham Yoga-in-the-Parks Tour, now an annual event in its 2nd year.

Shortly after the publication of this book, we will hold our first 50-hr. Kaleidoscope Community Yoga advanced intensive teacher training program at Inspire Studio, run by Ruby Koa, also in Bellingham, WA.

And where it will go from there, only time will tell. We invite you to be a part of it.

INFLUENCES

The most formative influences on Kaleidoscope Community Yoga, (besides the project itself and the students) have been my own studies and experiences of: water, mathematics, philosophy, nature, wildlife, patterns, designs, textures, and sacred geometry. The most formative somatic influences on Kaleidoscope Community Yoga have been my own studies and experiences of: 5 rhythms, contact improv, modern dance, swing dance, square dance, contra dance, tango, rueda de casino, various kinds of folk dancing, ballet, shintaido, aikido, tai chi, qi gong, yoga, kung fu, healing dance aquatic massage, and thai massage. Qi gong, yoga, and thai massage, in particular, have honed my sense of the body and the possibilities of movement, and have contributed strongly to my sense of a deep, thorough, liberating, opening systematic treatment of the body. Contact improv, in particular, has freed my mind from contextual associations and encouraged more interesting combinations of bodies. And square dance, contra dancing, and rueda de casino, in particular, have helped serve as models of different forms of group calling, naming, sequencing, movement, and organization. Healing dance aquatic massage has also helped inform my sense of shared dynamic energy and how to develop a working, coherent system of levels and names with concrete images, and how to describe things.

VISION

In any case, as the world gets more and more populated, the ability, and the art, of sharing and getting along with one another will only become more and more important. I do truly believe that combining the depth and wisdom of the roots of the ancient traditions of yoga and transforming it and re-understanding it as a shared social, communal activity will be a major new direction of infinite potential growth for yoga in the new millennium.

And I believe we are just at the very beginning of the very tip of the iceberg, so to speak, for the kinds of huge and amazing collective yoga poses we will see in the future.

And I invite you to join us.

LIST OF SYNONYMS AND NAMES FOR COMMUNITY YOGA

Community yoga
Synchronized yoga
Sacred circle yoga
Group yoga
Collective yoga
Social contact yoga
Mandala yoga
Group process yoga
Group mind yoga
Group field yoga
Group energy yoga
Energy field yoga
Collaborative yoga
Sharing yoga
Pattern yoga
Universal yoga
Mathematical yoga
Sacred geometry yoga

FUN, IMAGINATION, AND CREATIVITY

Kaleidoscope Community Yoga is about people.
About connecting with them, and getting to know them.
And there are as many ways to do that as you have time and interest for.
In addition to the classic Kaleidoscope shapes presented in this book, there are an infinite number of possibilities for unique, irregular, and unusual poses, shapes, and combinations...
Here we present just a few to inspire you...

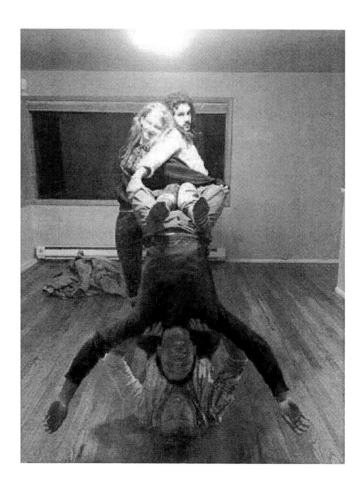

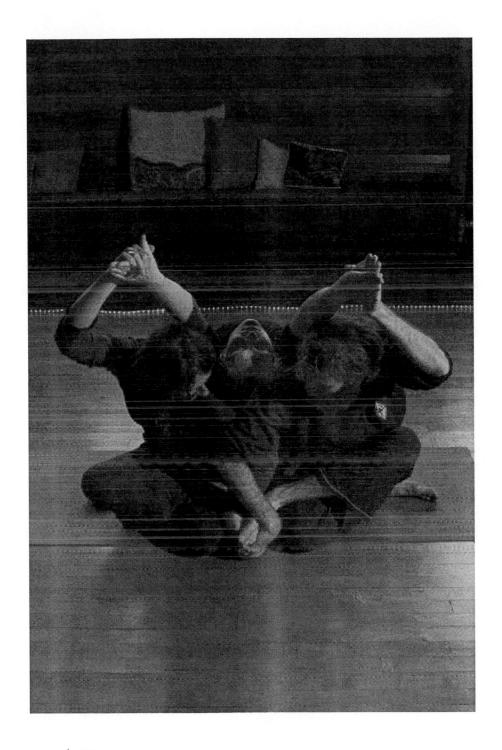

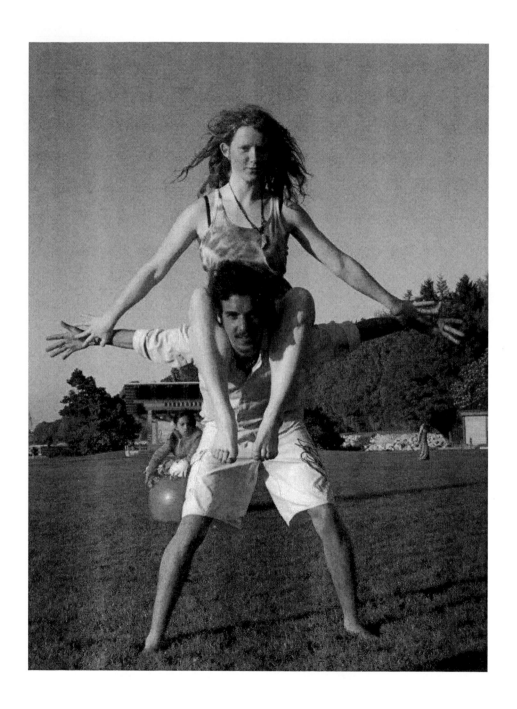

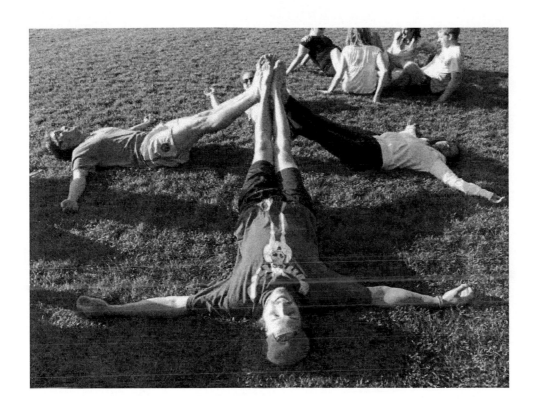

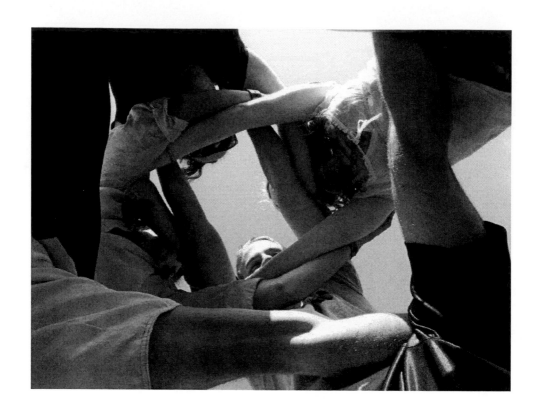

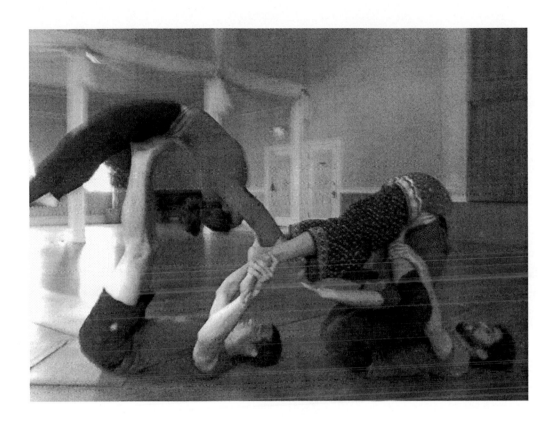

And, perhaps most important of all, don't forget to have fun...

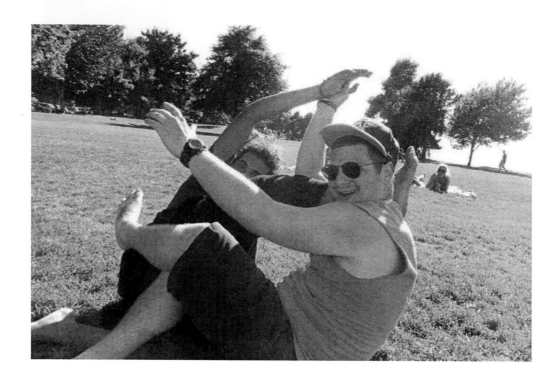

INDEX

D

knees, hands to knees baddha konasana clover (level 5) #45... p. 117

L

R

S

T

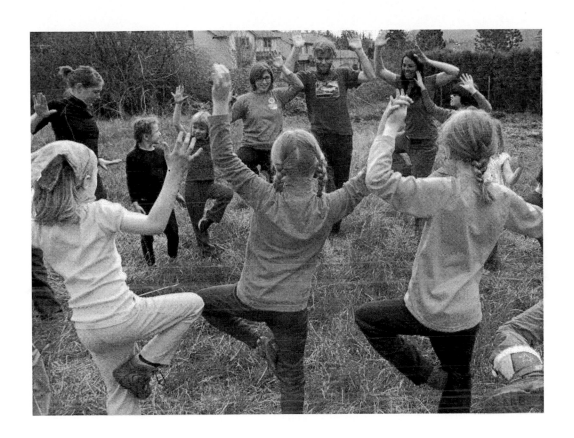

Pose credits:

Sandra Amiry, Brian Anderson, Rachel Arnold, Nikki Bacon, Becca Barbanell ("Dreamyball Dang"), Mimi Beeson, JC Beiting, Jae Bergeron, Jill Beringer, Briana Berkowitz, Cheyenne Black, Danielle Bois, Ken Bothman, Cassidy Bristol, Paige Brummett, Jamie Busch, Bodiye Cabiyo, Erica ("Lilly") May Carey, Christie Cassel, Angie Charette, Jesse Charette, Sara Charette, Eric Cole, Sherry Cornelius, Lydia Cotton, Judith Culver, Gina Curwick, Jaleh Davari, John Dean, Nikolette Deloge, Chris Dion, Stephanie Dougherty, Douglas Drake, Scott Draper, Joseph Ecklund, Frances Erickson, Link "Littlepaw" Falsetto, Nate Fine, Amanda Folsom, Adam Gaya, Carly Gilder, Bryan Givens, Ladina Gmur, Jonathan Gore, Mary Gossard, Susan Grace, Nat Hagood, Ali Hancock, Marren Hanna, Rylee Harlow, Ben Harris, Isaac Hart, Annie Hewlett, Carly Heying, Sander Hicks, Desirae Hill, Jenny Hoang, Cassandra Hogl, Patrick Holahan, Spruce Horowitz, Christiane Hueglin, Mason Hughes, Larry Hurvitz, Dimitri ("Mimi") Irish, Peter James, Cara Jerde, Maura Jess, Lauren Jones, Skyler Jordan, Kathryn Joy, Tessa Juhl, Kelly Kelsey, Renee Kennedy, Evan Kerl, Erin Kidulson, Tee King, Jean Kroll, Kate LaSpina, Mischa Levine, Oscar Lichtenstein, Melanie Lum, Isabel Machuca-Kelly, Mehdi Makraz, Gabriel Mannino, Ran Mapps, Reed Mcintyre, Nancy Metcalf, Melissa Miller, Alborz Monjazeb, Olivia Moon, Burke Mulvany, Makenzie Blake Mumford, Dan Nagy, Lo Nathamundi, Megeara Noland, Brian Norvaisis, Linda Ost, Tsena Paulson, Alex Peregrina, Mai Peregrina, Maya Peregrina, Alejandro Quezada, Caitlin Quigley, Jordan Rain, Stephanie Rambo, Danny Ray, Ezra ("AJ") Ritchie, Marlene Riviere, Kelly Robbins, Yuri Rostykus, Haley Rutherford, Phoenix Sage, Aldo Schipper, Stephanie Scott, Mario Sheldon, Phimpha Simongkhonh, Devin Singh, Sarahope Smith, Lillian Soderman, Dannie Soloff, Arielle Spayd, Jenni Spicer, Tara Stanley, Jill Sturdevant, Julie Thompson, Leah Thomson, Marc Tobin, Arisana Tolomei, Suzanne Tom, Sam Top, Beila Ungar, Molly Van Hart, Jesús R. Velázquez, Rose Vogel, Jayson Wagner, Andy Wargo, Charissa Waters, Ed Welter, Jeffrey Westcott, Noah Young, Curtis Yu, Yahya bin Yutte, and many others and more to come.

Photo credits:

Teddy Anderson, Briana Berkowitz, Christie Cassel, Sara Charette, Heather Dalberg, Bryan Givens, Jaime Hernandez, John Hogl, Eero Johnson, Jorge Lausell, Mehdi Makraz, Alborz Monjazeb, Lo Nathamundi, Alex Peregrina, John Rentschler, Phoenix Sage, Jill Sturdevant, Molly Van Hart, Aidrien Wilkins, Kendyl Zillich, and many others and more to come.

EPILOGUE

See you in the shapes.

Blessings.

Lo

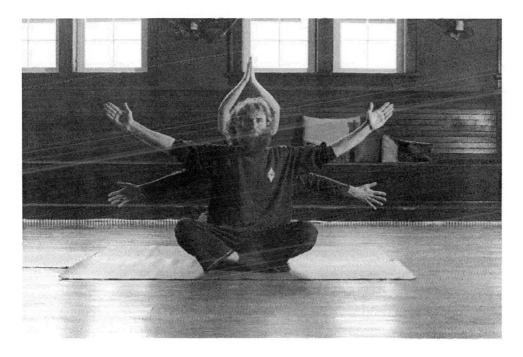

www.kldyoga.org

Ideas?
Feedback?
Appreciation?

We would love to hear from you.

Hold us fondly in your thoughts. Write us a letter. Send us your photos. Call on the phone. Come and visit. Come find us at a festival. Or invite us to your city, town, or remote natural setting for a workshop or a training. Really. No matter where you live.

We love that.

We do all sorts of gigs, trainings, classes, workshops, festivals, weddings, parties, special events, etc.
Please contact us if interested.

For full-color artbooks, limited edition copies, spiral bound copies, copies in various languages, wholesale orders, educational discounts, library orders, electronic copies, and other book inquiries, feel free to contact us.

We also welcome all media inquiries about the project.

For shirts, stickers and other merchandise, and all other orders and inquiries, please contact us directly at the contact info listed below.

info@kldyoga.org
loswirlingwaters@gmail.com

(360) 676-1487

Lo Nathamundi
Infinite Designs
Kaleidoscope Community Yoga
3628 SE 13th Ave.
Portland, OR 97202